From Struggle to Strength

A Father's Journey with Autism and the Power of Hope and Positivity

Harry Psaros

Aurora Corialis Publishing

Pittsburgh, PA

Disclaimer

The author is not a medical professional. He makes no claims to diagnose, treat, cure, or prevent any condition or disease. This book is meant to serve as an educational tool for the reader. Please consult with your doctor if you have any questions about starting a new supplement, exercise, therapy, treatment, or herbal regimen.

The advice and strategies found within may not be suitable for every situation. This work is sold with the understanding that neither the author nor the publisher is held responsible for the results accrued from the advice in this book. This book is not intended as a substitute for consultation with a licensed practitioner.

Although the publisher and the authors have made every effort to ensure that the information in this book was correct at press time and while this publication is designed to provide accurate information in regard to the subject matter covered, the publisher and the authors assume no responsibility for errors, inaccuracies, omissions, or any other inconsistencies and herein and hereby disclaim any liability to any party for any loss, damage, or disruption caused by errors or omissions, whether such errors or omissions result from negligence, accident, or any other cause.

Use of this book implies your acceptance of these disclaimers.

Praise for From Struggle to Strength

"As an educator and owner of the Brain Balance Center in Pittsburgh, Pennsylvania, helping families and children overcome struggles is my true calling and passion in life. Breakthroughs are possible, and Harry Psaros reminds us of this in his book, *From Struggle to Strength*. His book presents honest and practical guidance for parents with children diagnosed with autism. However, it is truly written for any parent with a child who is struggling. Sharing his personal experience as a father, Harry provides words of wisdom to parents who need encouragement, support, and a dose of optimism. Even if we do not have a child who struggles, *From Struggle to Strength* is a good reminder for us all that we can overcome obstacles by tackling them with courage, positivity, and resilience."

–Megan Galando, M.Ed, Owner and Executive Director of the Brain Balance Center of Wexford

———

"*From Struggle to Strength: A Father's Journey With Autism and the Power of Hope and Positivity* is a truly empowering and inspiring book. It tells the story of a family's transformation from 'Guess' to 'Gus,' as they navigate the challenges of raising a child with autism.

"The book beautifully captures the father's perspective and his unwavering determination to provide the best possible life for his child. It delves into their struggles, the emotional rollercoaster they experience, and the obstacles they overcome along the way.

"What makes this book truly remarkable is the author's ability to infuse every page with hope and positivity. Through his storytelling, he not only shares valuable insights into autism but also emphasizes the power of love, resilience, and unwavering support.

"Reading *From Struggle to Strength* left me feeling inspired and uplifted. It is a testament to the strength of the human spirit and a reminder that with determination and positivity, we can overcome any challenge. This book is a must-read for anyone seeking hope and encouragement in the face of adversity."

–Katie Harrill, Creative Arts Supervisor and Music Therapist at Wesley Family Services

———

"Harry shares his honesty, doubts and fears in *From Struggle to Strength*. You will laugh, cry, and be encouraged by his family's journey as they navigate ASD. Harry and his determined family prove that with the right support, challenges can become joys to celebrate."

–Kelly Cain, Founder of Autism Caring Center

———

"*From Struggle To Strength* gives fathers of special needs children the connection and understanding that is not always readily available to them. But the book also encourages moms to pause; it gives us a lens to see the male perspective more clearly.

"As a mom of a special needs child, Harry's story made me realize that I did not take enough time to consider how Dad was handling things. We all just become so busy with the schedule autism brings. Thankfully Harry has so bravely taken the time to share his experiences with his son Gus.

"Harry is a true contender against the relentless opponent we call *autism*. It bobs and weaves, but Harry reminds us, in an incredibly positive and powerful way, that we too have all the right moves. This book, no matter where you are in your journey, will be the encouragement you need in your corner of the ring!"

–Carrie P. Holzer, Autism Mom and Author of *Building Puzzles Under Water: An Autism Story*

———

"A must read for any family touched by autism, but especially for a 'warrior' father who may be struggling and needing a boost of strength from another father's journey.

"Harry Psaros writes about the roller coaster of having a child with autism. From denial to acceptance and then to thriving, Harry's rawness and positivity gives insight and hope when times may feel hopeless and helpless as a parent with a child with special needs.

"His story, Gus' story, is heart wrenching, captivating, and empowering all in one. This book is a guide to helping yourself, your family and your child. It gives real-life trial and error examples and concrete suggestions of how to help you and your child continue to move forward and live their best lives '2% at a time.' The energy and positivity are inspirational and contagious! This book will forever be in my library of resources for families. "

–Patty Maxwell, Owner of Engage Kidz LLC

Dedication

I dedicate this book to my late father, George, a beacon of guidance and the epitome of strength. Thank you for painting the picture of greatness in fatherhood. Your every sacrifice has etched a story of love in my heart, inspiring me to reach for the stars while staying grounded in your invaluable teachings. May your memory be eternal.

Acknowledgements

Michelle, thank you for lighting my world with your radiant smile and heart. I don't tell you often enough how much you mean to me. You are my soulmate, my best friend, my home. I love you to the moon and back. You are my happy place.

Mom, words cannot express how grateful I am for your unwavering love and support. You have been my foundation—my biggest fan—cheering me on every step of my life. There is no better *yia yia*. I love you with all my heart.

My brother Michael, without you, this book would still be a dream tucked away in my heart. You have always been and will always be my hero. Your support made it possible for us to explore every option for Gus. Your compassion means the world.

I want to express my deepest gratitude to my incredible extended family for always being there when we needed you most. Your unconditional love and unwavering support gave us the strength to push through even the darkest days. You were the lighthouse guiding us home, the shelter in the storm, our rock in moments of distress. Our family may be small, but we are mighty.

Thank you, Sarah Gorry, for your mentorship, guidance, and patience with me throughout the writing process. You will forever be my official Book Yoda from the United Kingdom.

Thank you to the heroes who guided Gus along his journey. To the teachers who nurtured his young mind, the therapists who unlocked his potential, the principals who advocated for him, and the physicians who cared for his wellbeing—your compassion and dedication made all the difference.

Table of Contents

Introduction

"Choose to be optimistic, it feels better."[1]

– Dalai Lama

People with autism spectrum disorder (ASD) cannot predict how their lives or condition will progress. Unfortunately, I have encountered many parents, particularly fathers, who jump to conclusions about what their child's life will be like, and it's not a very positive picture. The truth is, every person, including those with autism, continues to grow, evolve, and flourish throughout a lifetime.

Who am I to speak on this subject? My name is Harry Psaros. I am your everyday type A, proud Greek, sports fanatic. In my professional life, I am an executive neuroscience account specialist developing therapeutic BOTOX® clinics with an emphasis on migraines.

In my community, I am president of the North Fayette Township's parks and recreation board and VP of All Saints Greek Orthodox Church in Weirton, W.Va. Known as "The Pitt Guru"—a top social media influencer for University of Pittsburgh athletics—I am also the senior writer for *Pittsburgh Sports Now* (a digital news platform).

---

[1] Dalai Lama XIV, Goodreads, Retrieved December 19, 2023. https://www.goodreads.com/quotes/67749-choose-to-be-optimistic-it-feels-better.

As for my personal life, I have the privilege of being the husband of a strong, beautiful, superhero of a woman who is a key player in this story—Michelle. I have a lot of titles to my name, probably too many, but there is one title that is easily my favorite: Dad.

I am the proud, proud father of two sons, Gus and Max ... and I am also a battle-tested, well-read dad of a child on the autism spectrum.

One of my final titles includes being on the board of directors for The Autism Caring Center (Canonsburg, PA) and one of the founding families of North Fayette PALS (Providing Assistance, Love, and Support), an organization for special needs children.

In 2014, I had the honor of speaking at The Autism Notebook Connection Conference in Pittsburgh. After I finished giving my speech, I noticed a line of women forming—*five, six, seven*. I did not know what was going on, but as I spoke with them, it became evident. Behind each mother, there was a resistant father back at home. Each woman lined up to ask me, "Can I have your cell phone number?", "Can you call my husband?", "Can you talk with him?"

I soon came to realize, unfortunately, there is major resistance in fathers to assist their children on the autism spectrum. I am not saying all fathers are resistant, but far too many are unwilling to accept their child's diagnosis due to stubbornness or a macho attitude. I can say this because I was that guy, but I am not anymore. I want dads to learn from my mistakes so they can help in the successful development of their child on the spectrum. All resistance does is create distance between husband and wife and between parents and their children ... and that's the last thing an autistic child needs. What's needed is unity—mom and dad working together and in their child's corner, fighting for them.

There are a multitude of books written by amazing, warrior moms of children on the autism spectrum, but there are very few from a father's perspective. (Believe me, I know because I blew through three audio books a week and have a shelf of over 30 books on autism.) And that is exactly why I am writing this book ... to be that voice for dads everywhere. While I might not be able to call every father and speak with him personally (though I'd love to!), hopefully, I can reach them through telling my story—Gus's story.

Even if Dad isn't the one holding this book right now, or adding this to his Amazon cart, my hope is that this book will be a tool for anyone reading it. Maybe it's you—the badass, warrior mom—reading it. If so, leave it open on your husband's desk, highlight key points, or slap it directly in his hands and say, *OK, Jackass, read this chapter, three pages, a sentence, whatever. Just see if this sinks in.* Gus may not be *your* son or daughter, but I believe through his story we can provide hope to parents and children suffering.

This book is not another "how to" book attempting to describe a clearly delineated path to improvement for your child because no two children on the autism spectrum are alike. I will be sharing plenty of practical advice for nurturing your child's growth, but I will also be diving into the attitudes and mindsets that are keys to success. As the John Addison quote goes, "You've got to win in your mind before you can win in your life."[2] My goal is to provide you with both the mental frameworks and actionable steps to help you and your child thrive.

---

[2] John Addison, Goodreads. . Retrieved December 27, 2023. https://www.goodreads.com/quotes/11482709-you-ve-got-to-win-in-your-mind-before-you-win

Chapter 1: Where It All Started: Gus's Story

"Be like a flower, survive the rain, and use it to grow."[3]

– Unknown

When you find out you are expecting your first child, you have this assumption that you will be the proud parents of a *normal*, happy, and healthy baby. You are so caught up in the excitement of what is to come that no one—*no one*—thinks about autism when they see that positive pregnancy test. As I held my newborn son for the first time, autism was not even on my radar. I was dreaming about this journey we were about to embark on as a family and all the things I was going to teach him as he grew up.

I thought back to all the things my parents taught me: the importance of a firm handshake, looking people directly in the eye, speaking to elders first as a sign of respect, being non-judgmental, treating everyone with kindness, the art of public speaking, and using proper grammar. I reflected on living with positivity. (I do not "do negative.") As well as having self-confidence, abiding by my mantra, *strong body, strong mind*, and taking impeccable care of my health through nutrition and exercise. I live by the famous Bruce Lee quote, "Optimism is a faith that leads to success."[4]

---

[3] Unknown, https://medium.com/@brian.ford/be-like-a-flower-survive-the-rain-but-use-it-to-grow-bfba498e9235#:~:text=So%2C%20.
[4] Bruce Lee, "Great Bruce Lee Quotes," Sources of Insight. https://sourcesofinsight.com/bruce-lee-quotes/.

I even had a running joke with my friends that my wife, Michelle, and I were having the University of Pittsburgh's next great linebacker. As it turns out, Gus's life panned out differently than either of us expected.

Gus was a sickly child, and we were in and out of the hospital all the time. He was constantly on steroids and antibiotics to treat his chronic ear infections, neither of which he should have been on long-term. The antibiotic destroyed his gut biome, which is critical to brain development, but our child was sick, so we felt like we had no other option. He was even sick at the time of his vaccinations, and they still blasted him with four to five vaccines at once!

I realize there is a lot of controversy around this topic, and I am not going to say, *All vaccines are bad!* No, I am not stating that at all. Not all vaccines are bad, they save lives. What I do believe is that the physiology of children on the spectrum is different. I have had discussions with countless parents of children on the spectrum—almost all of them point to the period after the MMR vaccinations as the slippery slope that exacerbated their child's ASD symptoms.

I am not a physician, but I have done copious amounts of research and sat through a multitude of lectures, and I believe many children with ASD experience immunoexcitotoxicity during this time frame. What happens is an ugly cascade of events that eventually leads to the degradation or alteration of the child's brain. Oxidative stress and inflammation lead to microglial activation which leads to excitotoxicity, then eventual neurological degeneration. [5]

---

[5]Russell L. Blaylock, "Why immunoexcitoxicity is the basis of most neurodegenerative diseases and systemic immune activation: An analysis," Surgical Neurology International,

Let me explain further, children with ASD lack adequate amounts of glutathione, which assists in detoxifying many harmful toxins in their system—chemicals, metals—and eliminates excessive glutamate. The depleted glutathione leads to higher levels of glutamate in the brain, triggering events that disrupt typical brain function.

In layman's terms, if glutathione is Batman, glutamate is the Joker. You have allopathic physicians saying, *No, no. That is not the case. You are wrong*, but what the autistic community is trying to say is, *We know our kids react differently.* There are so many kids on the spectrum with weak immune systems, so the vaccines need to be spaced out. Do not give five at once! I think that is what parents want the doctors to understand. But I digress.

Gus was our first child, so we did not have any *normal* childhood behaviors to compare his with. (When you have your first child, you do not know what you do not know.) However, after Gus received his dose of the MMR vaccine at around 18 months, Michelle started noticing her best friend's child doing all these things that Gus just did not do. He would not respond to his name being called and was indifferent when Mom or Dad left the room.

In those days, Michelle was a nurse. She was working 12-hour shifts, three days a week. When she dropped Gus off at my parents' house to go into work, he could have cared less that she left. Normally, a child at that age reaches for Mom, or cries, *Mommy, don't leave!* With Gus, there was never any of that.

My wife voiced her concerns to the pediatrician only to be met with, "Oh, he is just a boy." OK, but this boy was not talking like the

---

https://surgicalneurologyint.com/surgicalint-articles/why-immunoexcitoxicity-is-the-basis-of-most-neurodegenerative-diseases-and-systemic-immune-activation-an-analysis/.

other boys did. "Boys sometimes talk late, don't worry about it." Fast forward to three years old, Gus was still not talking in complete sentences. When he did start speaking, it was in what's called an echolalic speech pattern. It was almost like a parrot mimicking your speech pattern. I would say, "Hi, Gus!" and he would say, "Hi, Dad!" I would ask, "How are you?" and he would echo back, "How are you?" We started picking up that a conversation with him was predicated on what you asked him, but it stopped there. Again, Michelle voiced her concerns but was met with resistance.

Once preschool started, Michelle noticed the telltale sign: Gus would not socialize with the other kids. She was adamant that something was not right, but nobody else was seeing it. At the time, she was not even trying to say that Gus had autism. Back then, we did not even know what it was. There wasn't this mass knowledge of autism like there is now, but in her gut, she knew that something was not right.

No matter how hard she tried to get others to see it, no one was grasping what she was saying. Everyone, including family and "friends," would say, "He is fine!" Even the pediatrician was telling Michelle not to worry. It was as if they were looking at my wife thinking, *Oh, she is a little bit crazy,* as if she was a hypochondriac or had Munchausen syndrome by proxy.[6] (That's when people lie that someone in their care is sick to get sympathy or attention.) Even the one person my wife should have been able to lean on, back her up, and say, *You are not crazy,* (*ME!*) was blind to it.

---

[6] Factitious Disorder (Munchausen Syndrome by Proxy): What Is It & Symptoms (clevelandclinic.org).
https://my.clevelandclinic.org/health/diseases/9834-factitious-disorder-imposed-on-another-fdia

Instead of having her back, I was angry. *Why label our son? Maybe he is simply introverted?* I am the type of guy who runs on positivity. I could have fun at an insurance seminar! Michelle often sees me grinning like a butcher's dog because I love to laugh, and I constantly have a smart-ass comment or funny quip in my back pocket. (I put it down to having watched too much Monty Python.) It was too hard for me to believe that a guy who many claim *energizes a room* could have a son with a condition that robs him of social skills. You could call it a "not *my* son!" moment.

He was *my boy*, so my assumption was that he would be the guy who owned every room he walked into. Like father, like son. In my mind, having a child who struggled to meet others socially and make his presence felt wasn't part of the plan. We were going to have a football hall-of-famer, for goodness' sake! It was impossible for me to grasp.

Michelle, though? She persisted. Her mommy's intuition kicked into full gear, and she was adamant something was wrong with our son. Warrior moms, true badasses, know how to cut through the chaos and frustration. Almost the exact month that Gus was diagnosed in 2007, Oprah had a big special called, "Faces of Autism," that was held in conjunction with Autism Speaks, the nation's largest autism advocacy organization.[7] That is when Michelle started to connect the dots: our son could be on the autism spectrum.

The straw that broke the camel's back was a preschool birthday party at a pizza place. When Michelle and Gus arrived, all his classmates were seated at the table, eating pizza and playing games. Gus never made it to the table. They barely got inside the door. He banged on every surface and window he could reach like a bongo

---

[7] "Living with Autism," Oprah.com. https://www.oprah.com/world/living-with-autism/all

drum, going around the perimeter. At the time, Michelle thought, *Oh, my goodness! This is not normal*, but we now know Gus was stimming.

Almost all children and adults on the autism spectrum express some form of stimming. Stimming or "a stim" is a self-stimulatory behavior that involves repetitive movements or sounds. The most common are arm flapping (almost universal), rocking back and forth, spinning in circles, snapping, briskly moving their fingers, rapid blinking, and/or walking on the tips of their toes. Although stimming is often directly linked to autism, you do not have to be autistic to stim. When people are nervous, they tap their feet, bite their nails, and twirl their hair. That is a form of a stim.

I often tell people that children on the autism spectrum have an invisible antenna. When too much stimulation hits the invisible antenna, the child will react by stimming. At that time, one of Gus's stims involved banging on objects—imagine pounding a bongo drum but doing it on *everything*. Looking back, when Gus walked into a loud environment filled with children his own age playing and screaming, it was a sensory tidal wave hitting his invisible antenna.

That is when his preschool teacher, Josie Urso (Miss Josie), who became a good friend of ours, changed everything.

"Come and sit with me. Let's talk." Miss Josie grabbed Michelle's arm, "I did not know how to approach this with you, and I do not want to offend you, but something is not right here. I really think Gus might be on the autism spectrum."

In that moment, my wife finally felt a sense of relief. Someone else saw it, too! The people around her told her she was crazy, and as her husband, I should have been her rock, but I just did not see it. That brief feeling of relief was soon met with the reality of wondering what we need to do next.

Michelle came home broken and upset. Her raw emotion and Miss Josie's words were like bright beams of light shining through an abyss of denial. It started to open my eyes. For the first time, I realized that Michelle may be on to something, and that I owed her an apology—a *big* one.

Another realization came when Michelle told me a jarring story of Gus's behavior at a recent party. She explained how all the kids were captivated by the party magician's act, but Gus was at the back of the hall staring at a fan. My son, with a large group of his peers, was the outlier. As I heard the story unfold, I recalled that Gus *did* act a bit abnormally the week before at my cousin Maria's party. Each child at the party got a pencil in his or her little treat bags. While all the kids wrote or drew, Gus just twirled and stared at the end of the pencil. Suddenly, it all made sense, but as that realization set in, it felt like I was hit with a right then a swift left, in boxing terms.

I recall, in my typical type-A, over-caffeinated style, jumping onto my computer and starting to educate myself on autism. I even hit several bookstores as well. (As I said, I probably own, and have read, at least 30 books on the subject.) This was the first time I thought it was worth investigating, but where do we go? There really wasn't anywhere around us that we knew to go to talk to anyone about it, but as luck would have it, everything kind of fell into place.

My cousin's sister-in-law, Francine, worked two hours away at the Centre for Autism at Cleveland Clinic in Ohio. When I say we lucked out, that is no exaggeration. The wait list to get into the clinic was *six months to a year!* Then, if you wanted to see a specialist, add another six to eight months to that. Imagine what it would be like for someone who was going through what we went through and watching their child decline during a six-month wait.

The situation with Gus was time sensitive. We needed to address it ASAP, and so Francine was able to get us in within a two-week period. She expedited that process by a year—maybe more—a true hero. (If she was at a cardiology department, we would have been toast.) We took the first trip to the Cleveland Clinic to be tested. We were initially told that it could take up to two weeks to get the results once you met with the clinician, but they called us the next day saying they had a definitive diagnosis and wanted to set up a time to meet. Two weeks later, Michelle, Gus, *Papou* (Greek, for my rock star father), and I drove up for the diagnosis. We went back to Cleveland within a week, and the results were confirmed: Gus was autistic.

We had the longest two-hour drive back to Pittsburgh. All I could do was process my thoughts. I realized that my loving wife had been 100% correct, and I felt *horrible*. For so long, I had been stubborn, blind, and belligerent. I said to myself on the way home, *That is going to change today.* I owed my wife an apology for the six to eight months prior; then my thoughts shifted to Gus. What did this diagnosis mean for him? What was his life going to be like? Was he ever going to go to school? Would he ever get married? I started going over all these things in my head, and I had to grieve the loss of everything I thought I was going to have, start anew, and move forward from there.

I had a wide range of emotions, but I knew I had to be strong. I will be forever grateful that we had my dad—Gus's best buddy—with us on that trip. Gus and my dad were sitting in the backseat. My dad kept Gus entertained, jam-feeding him cookies, and encouraged us the entire time, "We got this, Har. We got this. He is going to be fine." We needed the assurance and encouragement that we were all going to do everything we could to help Gus. My parents have instilled in me, and I instill in my kids, that life is about mindset. At some point on that two-hour drive, I felt a shift in my mindset from devastation to hunger.

As Chinese military general, philosopher, and writer, Sun Tzu, famously stated, "He will win who knows when to fight and when not to fight."[8] Those initial "not *my* son" thoughts took on a different perspective. This time, they were, not my son—we are going to be different. We are going to do everything we can to help him improve day to day, week to week.

If you are a father, you are likely going to try to be the tough guy. I attempted to stay stoic and positive, but it is OK to take some time to grieve and understand what's going on. But do not stay there. It is equally important to come back with ferocity and knuckle up. While the first half of our car ride, I was lamenting—thinking of Michelle, and Gus's future—the second half was a *hell, no!* mentality. The gloves were off, and it was time to fight. In boxing terms, Michelle and I were backed into the ropes, and it was time to punch back. I was ready to help my child.

I often refer to Sun Tzu due to my martial arts background. He states in *The Art of War*, "Know thyself, know thy enemy."[9] I found myself in a hyperadrenalized state—similar to the state I am in when I am boxing or sparring in a dojo. I saw autism as my foe. I knew I couldn't conquer or cure it, but Michelle and I refused to allow it to hold our son back in life. Knowledge truly is power. Again, *know thy enemy*. I would encourage you to do the same.

---

[8] Quote by Sun Tzu: "(1) He will win who knows when to fight and whe..." | Goodreads. https://www.goodreads.com/quotes/8707883-1-he-will-win-who-knows-when-to-fight-and
[9] Quote by Sun Tzu: "Know thy self, know thy enemy. A thousand battl..." | Goodreads. https://www.goodreads.com/quotes/861176-know-thy-self-know-thy-enemy-a-thousand-battles-a

I finally had that fighting spirit Michelle possessed all along. We were going to get Gus the help he needed, but we quickly ran into a wall. Gus was diagnosed in Ohio, and we lived in Pennsylvania. Had we lived in Cleveland, The Clinic could have given us a list of things to do, people to see, clinics to go to. Unfortunately, their resources were limited to Ohio. *What the hell do we do now?* If only there was a checklist of what to do—*Do this, then do that when you get back to Pennsylvania*—the two of us would have been right on it. But there was no guidance on where to go once we got back home.

That said, I am grateful we lived in Pittsburgh at the time. As it turned out, where we lived became a critical part of Gus's story and treatment. Michelle and I grew up 30 miles from Pittsburgh in Weirton, W.Va.—an old, sleepy, steel town. My friend, Brent Dragisich, encouraged us to check out a new development in Pennsylvania even before Gus was born. At the time, we had no idea how critical that move suggestion would be to our journey. Turns out, it was a *huge* step for our family. Had we remained in Weirton, I am not sure where Gus would be today. Compared to Pennsylvania, West Virginia was a wasteland when it came to autism treatment, although I have since heard that the situation has improved. Still, we had to do all the research on our own. *What services do we need? Who do we see? Where do we go?*

It was challenging, but a friend of ours stepped in to help. She happened to know someone who immediately called us and said, "You need to get the medical assistance card because in Pennsylvania, if you do not have that, you can't get any services. You can't do anything." That was step one and is what really got the ball rolling when it came to treatment. A woman we were put in touch with happened to have a child who was going through the University of Pittsburgh's Western Psychiatric Hospital (Western Psych), which turned out to be the best thing on the planet for Gus. Their wraparound services were life changing. For those unfamiliar with the term, wraparound services include a team of trained professionals that work with your child to help improve his or her behavior. Key members of the team can include a behavioral specialist consultant (BSC), a mobile therapist (MT), and a therapeutic staff support person (TSS).

We knew we were going to be faced with a lot. Gus was going to need occupational, speech, and feeding therapy, along with wraparound services. It was essentially a full-time job. We were told, "It is either you or her, but one of you has to be home." So, Michelle made the decision to quit her nursing position and stay home with Gus. (Side note: She truly is the most caring and selfless human being I've ever met. Michelle was born to be a nurse, but some things are more important.)

We first started applied behavior analysis (ABA) with Western Psych and would have a BSC and a TSS come to our home for six hours a day. The therapists would get to the house around 8:30 a.m. and stay until 11:30 a.m. There would be an hour break for Gus to eat lunch, and then the next therapists would come for the afternoon session. Some of those days were exceptionally painful.

We lived in a neighborhood packed with children, many of whom played on our massive Rainbow King Kong Castle swing set that Michelle bought while I was away on a business trip. During the assembly process, I discovered that it was money well spent. It was so large it attracted all the children in the neighborhood. While the final screws were being installed, kids from all around the block waited eagerly with their mothers—it looked like Lollapalooza behind our house! We became the epicenter of the neighborhood, and it was tough keeping Gus indoors for therapy while kids played outside. But I will say Gus was very good about doing his work. He knew what he had to do, and we did not meet a lot of resistance with him. He did not scream to go outside, but at the same time, we made sure to close off everything so he could not see what was going on out there. It was more distressing for us not to be able to let him play outside, which goes back to grieving the loss of what we thought our life would be like. But you cannot focus on that, or it is going to make you crazy and block your child's progress. I hate to say it, but you just have to accept it and think, *OK, this is what he has, and we need to do whatever we can to help him progress. We have to focus on what we can do, not on what we can't.* Therapists ultimately told us that the swing set was a brilliant move. All interaction was good interaction for Gus, and the swing set was like free therapy. When Gus was not working with his therapists, we encouraged him to spend just as much time outside playing with his friends. The interaction with our neighbors, all of whom are family to us, allowed us to educate them on Gus's therapy and autism in general.

In the summer of 2009, Gus started art and music therapy with Katie Harrell at Wesley Spectrum, which is the autism part of Wesley Family Services. (Katie Harrell is incredible. I still see her every year at the Autism Caring Center's massive Summer Fade Away Festival fundraiser.) Things were going well—*very* well. Gus had become proficient at playing the piano. His grandmother, Mary Ann, was a music teacher, and it was great to see him flourishing with an instrument. He was also making eye contact and starting to interact with everyone around him. Michelle and I were ecstatic! This was the summer before Gus started kindergarten, and he had actually been discharged from speech therapy. He had met all his goals, and it was amazing. He was a completely different kid from the one two years prior! Many felt that he was essentially now a neurotypical kid. But that all came to a tragic end.

It was an afternoon like any other as Michelle and Gus were getting ready to leave for his piano lesson. Except, on this day, Gus had put on his Crocs and walked down the steps before Michelle. What she did not notice was that Gus had slipped his foot into those dreaded Crocs with the one strap forward instead of around his ankle. As Gus was going down the steps, his foot slipped out, tripped him up, and he fell down a flight of wooden stairs. When Gus got up, he seemed fine. There were no tears, but within an hour he was acting *off*. Gus seemingly lost his ability to play piano, and within hours, he was a completely different kid.

After the fall, Gus was diagnosed with a concussion that robbed him of his progress and therapy overnight. It was like starting over again, and it was heartbreaking. When Gus tumbled down those stairs, our hearts shattered into a million pieces. In an instant, the bright little boy we had known vanished, replaced by a shell of his former self. For nearly two years we had poured our blood, sweat, and tears into helping our son on the autism spectrum make meaningful strides forward. With a single concussive blow, it was as if all that progress had been erased. We watched helplessly as Gus regressed at a frightening pace, losing skills it had taken months of repetition and positive reinforcement for him to acquire. Where words once flowed, now there was only silence. Routines he had mastered were now confusing and frightening to him. It was utterly devastating to see our child unraveling before our eyes—the emotional equivalent of having one of my fellow Tang Soo Do black belts roundhouse kick me in the ribs. Gus was just not the same. (In case you are wondering, I gathered every last pair of those wretched Crocs in the house. With shaking hands, I threw them in the trash, cursing their very existence. I still never want to see another pair as long as I live.)

That fateful fall did not just give Gus a concussion—it dealt a concussion to the hopes and dreams we held for his future. In those bleak days that followed, Michelle and I struggled to process our grief and dismay. At that point, it could have been easy for us to throw our hands up in defeat, but it was a matter of hitting the reset button. We had to go back to the same mentality we had after Gus's initial diagnosis. We just had to keep swinging, keep fighting, and keep helping him. Michelle and I had to refocus our love and amplify our determination. As dark as it was, we knew we could never give up on our boy. Dim as the light seemed, we clung to hope that Gus would find his way back to us once more.

The next days were filled with difficult decisions as we worked to help Gus recover. The specialists advised that we immediately cease his beloved music therapy sessions and all other extracurricular activities, allowing his fragile brain to rest and heal. Though it pained us to disrupt his routine, we knew we must follow the protocol. Gus would need total cognitive rest to give his injury the best chance of healing. Our journey together was far from over. His therapies continued, and we prayed daily for his full recovery. Though the road was long, we remained hopeful.

We went back to speech therapy and occupational therapy. Nutritionally, Gus was underweight, so he also started feeding therapy. Kids on the spectrum can be picky eaters. They might only eat beige foods, like chicken nuggets, French fries, and pancakes. All the things that are not good for them. For Gus, he would recoil if you put a vegetable on his plate or if his ketchup touched his chicken nuggets before he was ready for it. It was imperative that we expand his palate.

Atypical eating behaviors are found in the majority of children with autism, so expanding their palates through feeding therapy is vital for their health. Many of these children have extremely limited diets, consuming few, if any, fruits, vegetables, or other nutritious foods. Feeding therapists work diligently to gradually introduce new healthy foods in a positive, encouraging environment. With patience and persistence, therapists can successfully help children try foods they previously refused.

For an entire year, they worked on slowly introducing new textures one baby step at a time. At each weekly session, the therapist would have Gus try just one new food texture before sending him on his way. He always reminded us it was a marathon, not a sprint. Gus had a long journey ahead to become comfortable with different textures, but there was one comical exception to this: sushi. It occurred roughly three months into therapy. The day little Gus tried sushi for the first time was one for the record books. We were grocery shopping when he spotted the colorful sushi rolls and asked, "Daddy, what's that?" I told him it was sushi, though he hilariously called it "sookie." When he said he wanted to try the California roll, I'll admit I was skeptical. I figured the unique flavors and textures would be too much for him. But I thought, *Hey, what could it hurt?* I love sushi, so if he didn't eat it, it would be more for me! I grabbed a pack of sushi rolls, and we headed home. As soon as we got in the door, Gus ripped open the package and crammed a whole roll in his mouth. "Oh, wow!" he mumbled through a mouthful of rice, seaweed, and avocado. He proceeded to inhale all eight rolls in about 30 seconds flat. I was stunned! My little boy who primarily ate beige foods had discovered a sudden love for sushi.

When Gus and I visited the therapist the following week, the feeding therapist's jaw hit the floor when I told him the story. Sushi is a "texture bomb"' that he never thought Gus would try! His therapist continued to introduce new foods and textures throughout the year, but he would occasionally surprise Gus with a piece or two of sushi. Gus remains a sushi fanatic to this day. In fact, it is his favorite food.

Despite making strides with sushi, Gus still had feeding issues and a long way to go in terms of treatment. He also had disrupted sleeping patterns, gastrointestinal issues, chronic respiratory conditions (pneumonia and sinus issues), and echolalia (unsolicited repetition of utterances),[10] amongst other ailments. Through many recommendations, we found our way to Dr. Scott Faber, owner of

---

[10] Echolalia: What It Is, Causes, Types & Treatment (clevelandclinic.org). https://my.clevelandclinic.org/health/symptoms/echolalia

Developmental Integrative Pediatrics located at The Children's Institute of Pittsburgh, and believed he might actually have the answers and strategies to help our son. (At the time of writing this book, his practice is in Bridgeville, Pa.)

When Michelle called to book the first appointment with Dr. Faber, the nurse was so kind. "Tell me a little bit about Gus."

"Aside from the fact that he was always sick, he does not sleep. He only sleeps two hours a night," Michelle said.

Now, this wasn't your average fussy toddler who refused to take a nap. Gus had a peculiar sleep pattern. Around 11 p.m., he would doze off, but after just 30 minutes, his eyes would snap open, and he'd be wide awake. For the next six hours, Gus would obsessively turn the lights on and off throughout the house. He'd flip a switch, eagerly stare into the illumination, then abruptly shut it off again. This cycle repeated all night long, lights flashing on and off like a strobe. Michelle and I could only imagine what the neighbors thought of our nocturnal light show—they probably wondered if we needed an exorcism or were hosting an acid filled rave!

It was the early days of our careers, and Michelle and I were running on empty. As a nurse, Michelle worked grueling 12-hour shifts back-to-back, leaving her exhausted and sleep deprived. After barely catching a few winks (due to the all-night Gus light show), she'd drag herself out of bed to do it all over again. Meanwhile, I was an engineer with a lengthy commute. I would drive 45 miles to work in my bouncy two-door Ford Explorer Sport, often drifting off on the road only to be jolted awake when the SUV hit a bump. Fueled by caffeine and adrenaline, we were the epitome of the *walking dead*. Getting through our workday was punishing and required pure determination. As the sleepless nights dragged on, our once vibrant health began to wither away. Michelle and I went from a young, energetic, athletic couple to looking and feeling worn out by the relentless insomnia.

When Michelle, my parents, and I met with Dr. Faber, Gus walked into the office underweight, pale, and with dark circles under his eyes. Our first meeting was to discuss a potential care plan and schedule a large number of baseline tests to unearth what may be disrupting Gus's system. Michelle and I were well aware that Gus had a multitude of issues, and we were desperate to roll up our sleeves and fix them. Finding nothing would have been devastating. When we returned for the results of the tests, I still recall the nervousness going into that appointment. We sat back and held our breath as Dr. Faber said, "We've got a lot to cover." There were answers, and we were finally able to breathe a sigh of relief. "I can help Gus. We'll get him to thrive, function at school and with his peers, and eventually get him to college." Dr. Faber was the first individual to offer us something we did not have— *hope.*

Dr. Faber diagnosed Gus with pervasive development disorder-not otherwise specified (PDD-NOS); immune system dysregulation (having to do with the copper to zinc ratio), loss of tolerance to casein, gluten, and soy; encephalopathy; sensory processing disorders (sight and touch); sleep onset latency; mixed language disorder; and fine motor development coordination disorder.

Although this was a daunting list of items to conquer, we had many of the answers we were desperately seeking. Chris Howard, a former NFL running back, once stated, "Your destiny is forged in the fires of your determination."[11] Between Michelle, my parents, and me, we had a blast furnace of determination. Our goal was to

---

[11] Chris Howard, https://quotefancy.com/quote/1790584/Chris-Howard-Your-destiny-is-forged-in-the-fires-of-your-determination.

see Gus improve and have a bright future. We left determined to get started and nothing was going to stop us.

Things with Gus continued to progress when we got involved with Wesley WonderKids™ a brilliant program that taught him to interact with other kids and enhanced his social skills. Though the swing set in our backyard created a miniature version of this social interaction for Gus, with Wesley WonderKids, I never felt guilty about the fact that he would rather be outside on a swing set than inside with therapy—this program was play and therapy wrapped up in one.

The team at WonderKids was incredible. They arranged social activities for the kids, monitored their interactions, and worked with them during the process. When you pick up your child, they have a score sheet for you. It was fun to pick up Gus and find out how many interactions he had that day, or how he noticed a child using a toy incorrectly and helped them. They had a big check sheet, and Gus was hitting on all marks.

Any parent of a child on the spectrum worries that their child will be alone, so Gus's graduation from the program was a proud moment for Michelle and me. The team told us, "Gus has matured so much; he is becoming a leader amongst the group." Before Gus was officially diagnosed with autism, I had such a hard time accepting he might have a condition that robbed him of social skills, but here he was, with social and leadership skills emerging. Gus's graduation from Wesley WonderKids is still one of my greatest memories.

Gus was working well with Dr. Faber, the supplementation regimen he recommended was paying dividends, and Wesley WonderKids had greatly assisted Gus in social situations. It appeared that we had wind in our sails.

I started noticing Gus making a staccato guttural noise. We had noticed a considerable decline in stimming, but I wondered if we were once again losing ground. I immediately addressed it using techniques the therapists had taught me. This cat and mouse game of hearing the noises then attempting to correct them went on for weeks. I would be lying if I did not admit my palpable frustration. My goal was progressive improvement for Gus, and it felt like we were declining ... or at least stuck in neutral.

One day I heard Gus making noises, and I decided to observe him instead of attempting to redirect or correct him. I noticed a slight twitch in his neck every time he made the noises. It hit me like a bolt of lightning: he cannot stop making them. They were totally involuntary—he may have Tourette syndrome. One of my best friends, John Thomas (my brother from another mother), had Tourette's growing up, and I was very familiar with it.

I walked over to Gus and asked him, "Hey buddy, can you control those noises?"

He looked me right in the eyes and stated, "No, Daddy."

I knew I had to immediately speak with Michelle and have him tested. Yes, another trip to a specialist. Michelle and I eventually were able to secure an appointment with Dr. Robyn Filipink, a pediatric neurologist at the Pittsburgh Children's Hospital. Dr. Filipink was the director of the Tourette Syndrome Clinic. She confirmed during our appointment that Gus indeed had Tourette's. We had a lengthy discussion about therapy and medication to curtail the tics.

To quote Jim Morrison, the lead singer of The Doors, my brain was "squirmin' like a toad."[12] Autism already made social situations daunting for my son and now he has to deal with involuntary noises and movements. Yes, another *new normal*. We had no other option than to press on with positivity and grit, fighting for Gus.

In the midst of searching for every modality we could find to assist Gus, we opted to see a Defeat Autism Now! (DAN!) physician while still maintaining his therapy and regular visits with Dr. Faber. Even though Dr. Faber is brilliant, and all other treatments had been effective, we still wanted another set of eyes on Gus's situation.

Michelle and I drove to Ohio to see the DAN! physician who had a significant waiting list. (I no longer remember his name.) Needless to say, business was booming for him at the time; the DAN! concept was a new, hot commodity. When we finally met with the physician, he wanted a sizable number of tests—blood work, fecal collection, the works—the majority being out-of-pocket. Fortunately, we had the finances to pay for the tests. Unfortunately, years ago, assisting your child on the spectrum meant a significant outlay of money.

When we returned to hear the outcome of the bloodwork and fecal collection, the DAN! physician spoke with us for an hour, and it felt like he never took a single breath. He "prescribed" an endless number of supplements and creams—a regimen that was sizable, expensive, and felt like a blitzkrieg of items we had to get Gus to

---

[12] Densmore, J., Krieger, R., Manzarek , R., Morrison, J., & Scheff, J. (1971, June). Riders On The Storm [Review of Riders On The Storm]. Bruce Botnick/The Doors.

take throughout the day. Michelle and I left the appointment feeling like we had been cudgeled over our heads.

For several months, we attempted to comply with the DAN! protocol, but it simply became far too cumbersome. At the end the day, Gus was just a child, and it wasn't easy for him to ingest nearly 20 supplements a day—a few of them tasted and smelled vile. After only a few months, we decided enough was enough. DAN! was a swing and a miss, and apparently not only for us. The DAN! protocol was discontinued in 2011.

We did not let the negative experience with DAN! discourage us from seeking out modalities for our son. You win some, you lose some. Little did we know that we were about to discover some things about Gus that were definitive losses. Michelle called me at work and told me Gus had failed the school administered hearing exam. It seemed odd to me because he had passed their auditory exam for three consecutive years, but I initially did not think much of it. The teacher indicated he may be experiencing temporary issues with his ears, possibly an infection. Later that day, Michelle was able to secure an appointment with an audiologist. We would have to wait a little over a week to solve the mystery of the failed hearing exam. I was on my way to a meeting with a client when my phone rang. It was Michelle, and I could tell something was wrong. Her voice was a mix of sadness and shock. She was straight to the point, "Harry, you won't believe this, but Gus can't hear on the right side. There's nothing there. I was told he doesn't even have a right auditory nerve."

I thanked her for calling, pulled my car over, and immediately canceled my appointment with my client. I told them it was a family emergency. The news simply impaled my soul. If you are taking score, my son was diagnosed with autism and Tourette syndrome, and I just discovered he was unable to hear out of his right ear. I hit a breaking point. My body erupted with emotion. I started violently sobbing, and I pounded my dashboard. In the simplest of terms, I lost it.

My body needed to be cleansed of repressed emotion and the flood gates opened. After a cathartic, yet utterly painful, ten minutes of sobbing, I decided to have a conversation with God. I simply asked out loud, "Why? What is your plan with my son? Why shackle a child with so many difficulties?" I have a strong, quiet faith, and I thought it was only fair to have an open conversation with my maker. Suddenly, I thought of the words my mother, Mary Ann, and a few other *yia yias* (Greek for "grandma") at my church, had said to me. (Your average *yia yia* has Yoda-level knowledge, but with better baklava.) All of them told me, "God has a plan. Have faith." How could I ignore that advice?

I arrived home late that day and had practiced the pep talk I would give Gus. I did not want him to be devastated by the news. Michelle and I had a lengthy discussion. The audiologist explained that Gus would have a processing issue. There is a phenomenon known as "right-ear advantage."[13] Speech heard through the right ear reaches the part of the brain that processes it in about 20 milliseconds. The same speech heard through the left ear, however, takes between three to 300 milliseconds longer to reach the same part of the brain. Gus was only functioning with his left ear; therefore, his processing times were slightly delayed compared to his peers. When you are already talking about a child with social issues, this was a true liability.

That night I asked Michelle to let me put Gus in bed and have a heart-to-heart discussion with him. I was still emotional, but I

---

[13] *Is One Ear Better Than The Other?*, (2018, August 6), Nevada ENT, https://nevada-ent.com/is-one-ear-better-than-the-other/#:~:text=The%20phenomenon%20is%20known%20as.

wanted him to know that he would be OK. I started off the conversation tenderly, "As you know, buddy, the doctor told us you can't hear out your right ear. I want you to know that Mom and I will always be here for you, and you will be fine. You're my little champ."

Gus, with his infinite wisdom and positivity, looked at me with a grin and said, "Dad, what are you worried about? I can hear! I just heard what you said. I can still hear out of my other ear. I'm already fine!"

His words floated like butterflies and stung like bees. They knocked me straight out of despair and back on my feet. He not only took the diagnosis in stride, but he approached it with immense positivity. Your children can teach you lessons as well. I instantly started a cathartic chuckle. Gus joined in, and we laughed in unison.

"You're right buddy, you're going to be totally fine."

A left jab, right cross. Every fighter knows this classic one-two combination. Well, life decided to throw its own combination our way. The left jab landed when we discovered Gus was unable to hear out of his right ear. We reeled but stayed on our feet. We told ourselves it could be worse. Then life followed up with a crushing right cross.

Both of our sons struggled with persistent illness in their early years. Their hacking coughs were thick with gravelly mucus, which was alarming for us as parents. For years, we were told it was asthma. Gus was diagnosed with bronchomalacia (a condition that weakens the cartilage in the bronchi)[14] at one year of age. We

---

14 Bronchomalacia: Definition, Treatment & Causes (clevelandclinic.org). https://my.clevelandclinic.org/health/diseases/22771-bronchomalacia

thought maybe this was the primary problem, but his frequent illnesses continued. Both boys started nebulizer treatments, regularly inhaling albuterol mist to ease their wheezing. Gus eventually endured multiple sinus surgeries, and both boys underwent tonsillectomies and adenoidectomies. Despite the litany of procedures, our poor sons never seemed to fully recover.

We continued to combat frequent illnesses, some requiring antibiotics and steroids. While these drugs serve important medical purposes, research shows they can disrupt the natural balance of microbes in the gut. An imbalanced microbiome is linked to gastrointestinal issues and may exacerbate autistic behavioral symptoms.[15]

Michelle had a post-op visit with the ear, nose, and throat (ENT) doctor, and when she walked in with boys not looking well, the nurse gave her a befuddled look. She let Michelle know there was no way our sons should be displaying any severe illness after tonsillectomies and adenoidectomies, yet they stood in front of her with dark circles under their eyes and consistent, gravelly coughs. The wise, battle-tested nurse's intuition kicked in, and she strongly suggested Michelle take our sons to a pulmonologist. Michelle was able to secure an appointment with a prominent local pulmonologist within weeks.

The pulmonologist wanted to test for cystic fibrosis and primary ciliary dyskinesia (PCD). To rule out cystic fibrosis, our sons completed a sweat test. A sweat test is used to measure the amount of chloride in sweat. It's shown that children with cystic fibrosis can have two to five times the normal amount of chloride in their

---

[15] M.J. Tetel, G.J. de Vries, R.C. Melcangi, G. Panzica, S.M. O'Mahony, "Steroids, stress, and the gut microbiome-brain axis," *Journal of Neuroendocrinology* (October 2017), https://doi.org/10.1111/jne.12548.

sweat).[16] When the pulmonologist informed us that both passed the test and cystic fibrosis was ruled out, we were overjoyed.

The next series of tests were specifically for PCD. Our sons had to endure nasal scrapings, known as nasal brushing, and nasal nitric oxide measurements. Nasal scraping involves inserting a tiny brush into the nose to collect cells from the lining of the nasal passages. Not exactly fun, but necessary to examine the cilia under a microscope. Then comes the nasal nitric oxide measurement, which determines the levels of nitric oxide gas in the nasal cavity.

For this test, a small tube is placed in the nostril, and the patient must breathe normally for several minutes while the machine analyzes the breath. Again, not the most comfortable experience. Gus and Max displayed nothing but bravery throughout the uncomfortable procedures. Michelle received a call the day after the procedures were done from the pulmonologist. He stated, "I rarely make a call telling someone their child has PCD. To call someone and let them know that both their children have PCD never happens. Unfortunately, Gus and Max tested positive for PCD."

Learning that my sons had primary ciliary dyskinesia was a shocking and emotional moment. This rare genetic disorder affects the tiny hair-like structures that line the airways, making it difficult to clear mucus and prevent lung infections. PCD is estimated to occur in about 1 out of 15,000 to 20,000 people worldwide.[17] It all started to make sense. If their cilia were unable to remove the

---

[16] Cystic Fibrosis (CF) Chloride Sweat Test (for Parents) - Nemours KidsHealth. (n.d.). Kidshealth.org. https://kidshealth.org/en/parents/sweat-test.html#:~:text=The%20sweat%20test%20measures%20the

[17] Learn About Primary Ciliary Dyskinesia. American Lung Association. https://www.lung.org/lung-health-diseases/lung-disease-lookup/primary-ciliary-dyskinesia/learn-about-primary-ciliary-dyskinesia

mucus, no wonder they constantly had rough, gravelly coughs. Imagine what happens to a large metropolitan city when their garbage collectors decide to strike. The garbage piles up and the streets become congested. Gus and Max consistently had a thick buildup of mucus with no "garbage collectors" to remove it.

Suddenly, our lives changed as we scrambled to understand the diagnosis and treatment plan. Twice a day, Gus and Max had to throw on a vest that pulsated rapidly to help loosen the thick mucus in their lungs—similar to those used for COPD patients.

It broke my heart to see them struggle through the therapy, but over time, we saw improvements. The regular airway clearance significantly reduced recurrent infections, improved their breathing, and let them develop more normally. I distinctly remember looking at Michelle and asking, "When is the last time the boys were sick? Five or six months?" It was a miracle.

We had to explain to our sons that the vest treatments would be a lifelong endeavor. They had to make them a priority in their lives. Every six months the boys have their breathing capacity checked as well. Yet another lifelong practice they must adhere to. The plus side to PCD—remember, I'm a lunatic optimist—is exercise! The more the boys work their lungs, the better they can control their PCD symptoms. Those symptoms include chronic, severe respiratory disease and possible fertility issues.

When it comes to working out, Max is a total beast. You can find this guy in the weight room pumping iron 24/7. Football has turned him into a gym rat, obsessed with staying in tip-top shape. As for Gus, he's gotten on the health bandwagon, too. With help from his personal trainer and fitness guru, Bill Isenberg, Gus has traded in junk food for organic, low carb options. He's even swapped his couch-potato days for sweat sessions.

This journey has taught me how resilient children are and that even a serious diagnosis, like this one, can be managed with the right care and support. Gus was told he was deaf in his right ear then diagnosed with primary ciliary dyskinesia—he endured life's jab followed by the cross.

At that time, I reminded Gus of a Rocky Balboa quote about life (more on that later), "[...] it's not about how hard you hit, but how many times you can get hit and keep moving forward."[18] Gus was ready to move forward in life with the ferocity and grandeur of the iconic boxer Muhammad Ali.

Michelle and I were always looking for new methods to improve Gus's life, even if he only got 2% better. In 2013, I happened to catch an advertisement for Brain Balance®, a drug-free approach to improve brain function. There was something about it that gripped me, so I decided to call the local center. Brain Balance felt like something new and innovative, and, well, it turned out to be much more than that—it was life changing for Gus. Brain Balance is based on the work of Dr. Robert Melillo. Dr. Melillo wrote the books, *Disconnected Kids* and *Reconnected Kids*,[19] and he has convinced me of the power behind neuroplasticity. From the immense amount of reading I have done on the subject, in a nutshell, neuroplasticity is the nervous system's ability to reorganize its structure, functions, or connections in response to stimuli.

Every child on the spectrum is born with one hemisphere larger than the other. While that might initially look like an advantage, as the child grows and matures, that further separates the hemispheres, and there becomes a disconnect. What Dr. Melillo

---

[18] Rocky Balboa (2006) | It's Ain't About How Hard You Hit | MGM Studios. https://www.youtube.com/watch?v=kyQrl7AWeXg.
[19] https://www.drrobertmelillo.com/

and Brain Balance do is reconnect those synapses by enhancing the smaller, underworked hemisphere. As that happens, it is like a scale balances, tipping back up, and there is a reconnection. The reconnection I am referring to is a direct reference to brain plasticity, better known as "neuroplasticity." (Yes, you can reprogram your brain!) When you learn something new, your brain makes a new and improved synaptic connection. After reading Dr. Melillo's books, I dove into the book *The Brain that Changes Itself: Stories of Personal Triumph from the Frontiers of Brain Science*[20] by Dr. Norman Doidge. This book disproved that the human brain is immutable. I was further convinced that Michelle and I were making the right decision moving forward with Brain Balance.

To be clear, I do not work for Brian Balance or represent them in any official capacity. I am simply a parent sharing my experience. Now, some may dismiss Brain Balance as pseudoscience because of limited research supporting their approach. I understand that perspective, but here is my response: *it worked!* Their program was transformative for my son. Every child is different, of course. What I can say with certainty is that Brain Balance had an exceptionally positive impact in my son's case. The proof is in the results.

While I respect calls for more evidence, our family are firm believers based on the dramatic changes that we witnessed firsthand. The idea of dismissing Brain Balance and Dr. Robert Melillo's work entirely should give us pause. Doing so would be akin to rejecting the scientifically proven concept of neuroplasticity—the brain's ability to evolve, adapt, and grow new connections.

Just as our brains can create new neural pathways in response to experiences, so too can we foster greater balance and integration between its different regions. Neuroplasticity shows that our brains

---

[20] https://normandoidge.com/

are not static; they morph and change throughout our lives. So, let's keep an open mind to techniques that may support our whole brain functioning. With some effort, we can harness neuroplasticity to enhance brain harmony. The potential cognitive and emotional benefits make it worth exploring.

Gus began his first semester with Brain Balance. Each semester lasts three months, and the student is required to attend Brain Balance three times a week. During week one, the team hit the ground running. Gus was asked to complete a large questionnaire to determine which hemisphere he needed to work on during the semester. When we showed up, Gus was in what I would call an "autism fog." (I am sure every parent of a child on the spectrum can relate to this.)

When you are about to dive into 12 weeks of intensive brain work, you want your child to be *there*. Gus? He wasn't there. He was in his own little world. When they showed us Gus's responses to the questions, they were nonsensical. Some even infantile. His writing was way behind someone typically his age—it was very large and difficult to read.

Based on Gus's initial assessment, the Brain Balance team started a series of exercises to work on the side of the brain they needed to stimulate. For example, moving a pencil back and forth and following it with your eyes or using smells like coffee or cinnamon.

Between in-person sessions, the parents must facilitate the homework. You cannot just rely on other people to help your child—it must be a collective effort. I would say that anyone who is trepidatious about doing the exercises at home with their kids will more than likely fail, and it is not the program's fault. Complacency is death in this scenario. If the parents are not all in, it is not going to work. Will it be easy? Hell no! Look, kids are kids. They want to play; they want a break from everything. At times, it was taxing. Some days, Gus would fight us, but we stuck to the program.

Three times a week, Michelle would pick up Gus from Donaldson Elementary School in Oakdale, Pa. and drive roughly 40 miles to the Brain Balance Center located in the East Liberty neighborhood of Pittsburgh. If you are not familiar with the area, there is no easy way to get to East Liberty. You have to drive through the Fort Pitt Tunnels, make your way through the University of Pittsburgh campus (Hail to Pitt!), and then arrive at the center. The 40-mile journey could take well over an hour factoring in traffic. Why do I call Michelle a hero in this story? Because she is. I—along with my incredible parents, Mary Ann and George—would try to help as much as possible, but Michelle was the one who drove 240 miles a week through traffic. (That would be 2,880 miles per Brain Balance semester and a total of 8,640 miles to complete three semesters!) As luck would have it, less than one year after Gus finished with Brain Balance, a new center opened in Wexford, Pa., only 25 minutes from our house. The East Liberty Brain Balance is no longer in existence.

Another hero was Brain Balance's program director, Stephanie Domenico. She and her staff went out of their way to make us feel at home. Stephanie knew that we were driving Gus through the snarl of some of the worst Pittsburgh traffic and was always understanding if we were a little late or simply exhausted. (We are still connected to Stephanie to this day via Facebook.) When Gus got to the end of week 12, we were greeted by the team grinning at us. They slid a paper over to me, and I looked down and asked, "What is this?"

It was all of Gus's responses to the same questions they asked on day one. Only this time, they all made sense. Absolutely every question was answered correctly. Gus's penmanship was age-appropriate—it was no longer large, infantile, and difficult to read.

Not only that, but he was present in the moment. He wasn't in his own world talking about nonspecific things. Gus was *there*.

Michelle and I looked at this, and we were just blown away. At that stage, we signed up for two more semesters. By the end of it all, Gus had radically improved, and we did not have to add any pharmaceuticals. That is the other beauty of this program—you do not have to add anything to the body.

If you spend even a modicum of time with me, you'll hear me lecture about the importance of food consumption and lifestyle, not a temporary diet. There is nothing temporary about wellness and clean living. Brain Balance offered testing for Gus to discover food allergies and items that may disrupt him cognitively, so Michelle and I opted to pay for the testing. They offered something called the Brain Balance Diet, which consisted of eliminating highly processed snacks, sweets, and packaged foods in favor of lean proteins, fruits, vegetables, healthy fats, and whole grains.

After the work with Brain Balance, there was an amazing and evident shift in our son. Gus started advocating for himself. He started approaching his teachers if he had an issue. "I do not think I quite understood what you are saying on this equation," or "You marked this wrong, but I think the answer is correct." This time of self-assertion was not something you would get before—Gus needed assistance with everything.

One morning, Michelle and I had a meeting with all of Gus's Brain Balance teachers. As they each updated us on his progress, they were in tears. It was incredible to be surrounded by so many people who were not related to my son, working synergistically. People so invested in Gus, that they were crying while talking to us. Having finished their updates, they said, "He is done with us." Gus's three semesters of Brain Balance paid off—he no longer needed assistance in class.

I can only speak specifically about what worked for my son, but if you have a child on the spectrum, I encourage you to look at every modality available. (As I am writing this book, there could be a dozen new modalities out there.) Whether it is some sort of homeopathy, supplementation, or something like Dr. Melillo's work—as long as it is something that will not hurt the child, you have to be open to it. Do your research, and do not be shy to go beyond the lens of allopathic medicine. If we had not explored beyond the traditional allopathic path to improvement, I am certain Gus would not be where he is today.

Gus's journey has been an arduous one. After three grueling semesters of Brain Balance, our 17-year-old endured more struggles than most kids his age could ever imagine. At this point, Michelle and I faced a difficult decision—though it went against our nature, we chose to temporarily halt the endless search for new treatments. For once, we would allow Gus to simply enjoy the final years of high school. Sometimes knowing when to take a step back is just as important as pushing forward.

Gus needed time to recharge, and so did we. We wanted him to focus on the simple joys of family, friends, and schoolwork. College had long seemed an uncertainty, but by junior year, it finally became a reality. Through all the challenges, Gus persevered. He graduated from West Allegheny High School with a 3.8 GPA and ran with a close posse of friends. Mission accomplished. To this day, he continues to work out with his trainer, Bill, a gem of a human being. A girlfriend? We're not there yet! At the time of writing this book, Gus is a sophomore at Kent State University. He's a proud Golden Flash and has just signed a lease for a luxury apartment. The facility has a gym and pool. (*How did he pull this off, Michelle?*) On the way home from dropping him off at college, I went from depression to smiling, thinking of all that we've been through. It has been such a long, tough, arduous journey. But to see Gus flourishing, going off to college, and into a new chapter of his life is exciting. Of course, there is a big part of me that misses his constant presence at home—he is such a ray of sunshine. He always thinks positively and is so kind and bubbly. I call him my "happy hippie." He brings such a unique dynamic to the house, and I miss that. But man, oh, man—I am beaming with pride!

Was his freshman year a walk in the park? Far from it. There were some difficulties, but he made his way through. College has been a reminder that we'll always have challenges. With the exception of his close high school friend and roommate, Nick, most of Gus's friend group went elsewhere, and he found it difficult to meet people. At times, academically, he was overwhelmed. I believe it was God's way of telling us, *Remember, this is a marathon, not a sprint.*

One thing I will promise you: Michelle and I will remain in Gus's corner forever. We will do everything possible to see him succeed. Gus, in time, will make a positive impact on the world. Heck, he already has.

As for myself? My exploration into new modalities and supplements to assist Gus in his life's journey continues. I must agree with my fellow Greek, Aristotle, when he stated, "All men by nature desire knowledge."[21] I continue to obsessively study various cognitive therapies, such as nootropics, neuropeptide therapy, Brain SPECT technology, craniosacral therapy, and the list goes on. But more importantly, let me tell you about my partner in this journey, my wife, Michelle. I'll tell you a little secret: she loves the Quentin Tarantino movie series, *Kill Bill: Volumes 1 & 2.* Rarely does a violent action movie connect with her but Tarantino's masterful two-part revenge movie hit home.

---

[21]Aristotle,
https://www.oxfordreference.com/display/10.1093/acref/978019184373
0.001.0001/q-oro-ed5-00000434

The plot is straightforward: lead actress Uma Thurman is The Bride. She happens to be the deadliest female in the world and attempts to break free from the Deadly Viper Association Squad led by her former lover—Bill. The separation does not go well. The Bride is about to be married when the Deadly Viper Association Squad breaks into the church and attempts to kill her. She manages to survive and eliminates all her foes one by one. Her yellow and black one-piece jump suit in the movie is iconic. The Bride is a bad ass, a modern day Valkyrie. I believe Michelle could relate to Uma Thurman's character because she is equally as tough.

Throughout *Kill Bill*, nothing stops The Bride from achieving her goal. As the mother of a child on the spectrum, Michelle set her sights on doing everything possible to assist Gus to be the best that he could be, and nothing would stop her. Michelle is the personification of the warrior mom. I am honored to call her my wife and my son's mother. While The Bride accomplished her mission wielding a razor-sharp Hattori Hanzo katana, Michelle accomplished her mission with unrelenting love. Michelle and I cannot and will not rest in our pursuit to help Gus throughout his life.

Chapter 2: Words of Wisdom: Acceptance

"The Saint is a man who disciplines his ego. The Sage is a man who rids himself of his ego."[22]

– Wei Wu Wei

With autism, the goal of reaching "recovery" needs to get thrown out the window. The word "recovery" is wrong—your child can never "recover" from autism. What they can do is improve, and the gateway to improvement starts with acceptance.

It is imperative to accept that your child is on the spectrum and understand that the diagnosis equates to help, assistance, and improvement. It is understanding that your child is in a unique situation, one that is not going to go away. Acceptance is not just about your child. The path to improvement starts by unifying with your spouse and making sure you are both on the same page. (A healthy, self-assured man is there to support and elevate his child *and* his spouse—you have to do both.)

My wife and I often kayak around our second home in Bethany Beach, Del. There are great areas to kayak around South Bethany Beach and nearby Fenwick Island. We each have our own single kayak, and the thing about single kayaks is that they are easy to maneuver; in fact, you can get quite adventurous in them. I'd say

---

22 Wei Wu Wei, *Fingers Pointing Towards the Moon: Reflections of a Pilgrim on the Way*, (London: Routledge & Kegan Paul Ltd.), 1958, https://terebess.hu/zen/mesterek/fingers.pdf.

that Michelle and I are fairly skilled on individual kayaks and have little issue maneuvering them. However, on a recent trip to Bethany Beach, we opted to sign up for a guided tour and chose a tandem kayak. We had never attempted a tandem kayak before, but thought, *How hard could it be?*

Within 15 minutes of starting the tour in the waters of South Bethany, we quickly realized how difficult it was. Regardless of how hard we tried, we were unable to keep the kayak propelling forward in a straight direction—it would either veer left or right. It was frustrating and comical at the same time. Toward the end of the tour, we steadily improved. We were finally paddling in unison, and the kayak jettisoned forward.

What does this kayaking adventure have to do with autism, you ask? For your child to start improving, both you and your spouse have to paddle in unison. You both must accept the diagnosis, make a commitment to do everything possible to assist your child, and then move in the same direction. If you are both rowing in different directions, you are never going to go forward.

Are you going to have disagreements? Of course! Disagreements are natural in any relationship, but you must work to understand your spouse's different perspectives and be there to support one another. The key is understanding that even in disagreement, you are both working toward the same goals: assisting and helping your child improve. You and your partner need to work together synergistically.

Once you accept that your child is on the autism spectrum, you can shift your continual focus to improvement. That shift from a "problem-focused" mindset to an acceptance-mindset is what removes the angst, the arguing, the tension—it disengages the pressure. Acceptance removes all the undue stress and allows you and your spouse to focus on the child instead of the problem and move forward in unison.

Raising a child with autism can put immense strain on a marriage. Early media reports claimed divorce rates as high as 80% for these parents, though the data did not back that up.[23] The truth is less alarming, but still concerning. Studies show the divorce rate hovers around 30% for parents of children on the spectrum, significantly higher than average.[24] Caring for a child with autism requires round-the-clock effort that can leave parents exhausted and overwhelmed. Financial pressures also mount due to therapy costs and other expenses. The daily difficulties chip away at parents' overall wellbeing and relationship satisfaction. Many feel they lack adequate support. While the challenges are real, resilience is possible.

With understanding, patience, and access to resources, many couples mitigate autism's impact on their family. Some even report it strengthens their partnership. But there is no doubt this diagnosis tests a marriage like few others. Having one, or both, parents in denial, or apathetic, can be disastrous. Without acceptance, you will not only completely stymie the progression of your child, but there is the likelihood that you are putting extreme pressure on your marriage.

---

[23] Marina Sarris, Kenedy Krieger Institute, "Under a Looking Glass: What's The Truth About Autism and Marriage?," (April 2017), https://www.kennedykrieger.org/stories/interactive-autism-network-ian/whats-truth-about-autism-and-marriage#:~:text=The%20Myth%20of%20The%2080%25%20Divorce%20Rate&text=The%20researchers%2C%20from%20Kennedy%20Krieger

[24] Hartley, S. L., Barker, E. T., Seltzer, M. M., Floyd, F., Greenberg, J., Orsmond, G., & Bolt, D. (2010). The relative risk and timing of divorce in families of children with an autism spectrum disorder. Journal of Family Psychology, 24(4), 449–457. https://doi.org/10.1037/a0019847

You might be witnessing your child falling behind their peers, though you're doing all you can to help, but the person who is supposed to be in your corner—your spouse—is resisting every move you make. This pushback is harrowing.

When it comes to acceptance, men tend to be the most belligerent. (I do not want to make it sound like it is always the father who is not accepting—it is not—but it is common.) I've found that, oftentimes, men exude a testosterone-driven persona, where the father says, *Not my kid, he's just introverted.* (Hell, I was that guy!)

I once was asked to speak with a father whose son was severely autistic. Not only was he holding onto the not-*my*-son mentality, but he was also openly resistant to supporting his spouse. Their child was non-verbal, struggled with activities of daily living, and remained in diapers, yet the father seemed nearly oblivious to the situation. He was holding on to this not-*my*-son mentality, believing that things were going to improve. He had that bell curve mentality, thinking, *My son's on the other end. He is the alpha male leading the pack.* This father was lacking acceptance.

Bottom line: *You have to drop that ego, accept your child for who he or she is, and move forward toward improvement.* (Sadly, this father couldn't firmly grasp the scenario.)

If you continue to deny the diagnosis, even after your child has been evaluated by professionals, your child simply remains in the abyss. Your ego will hinder or eliminate the possibility of improvement. I've seen this error of intense male pride, or machismo, too many times when it comes to the diagnosis.

Let's face it. Every caring father wants to see his child succeed. He takes pride in his child's achievements—academically, athletically, etc. When your child receives an autism diagnosis, there is often this perception that he or she is now meek and will be labeled. My reply to that? Total bullshit. The truth is, if you accept the diagnosis and you love and nurture your child, he or she will find his or her own path. Even if a father does accept the diagnosis, there is still a tendency in a lot of men to think, *What are our options? What pill can we take?*

In the movie *Limitless*, starring Bradley Cooper, Cooper's character is a struggling writer facing unemployment and his girlfriend's rejection. His future looks bleak until he takes a pill that enables him to access 100% of his brain's abilities and transforms him into a financial wizard. That "limitless pill" is what a lot of parents of children on the spectrum are looking for, and it simply does not exist. I get it, believe me, I do. Every day I wake up and I wish I had a magic pill that I could give my son to rectify the situation.

Fathers want to fix things—it is in our DNA. The reality is, you can help your children, but you cannot fix them. Autism is something that your child is going to have for the rest of his or her life. You do not need a magic limitless pill, what you need is a change in mindset; one that says, *This is who my child is, I love him, and I am going to put together a path for improvement.* Our children are special, they are gifts. They may be on the spectrum, but they are not broken.

If you are struggling with acceptance, sometimes all it takes is a shift of perspective. When we were getting established with Dr. Faber, Michelle and I went to the Children's Institute of Pittsburgh. It was a humbling experience to be there. During the tour of the facility, I witnessed children with a multitude of severe disabilities—children who were handicapped. They were in wheelchairs, connected to countless tubes, and incapable of speaking. To see that really hit home. *What was I bitching about?* Shame on me! I had a son I could speak with and wrap my arms around. A son who, if I did my due diligence with my wife to help him, would have a future. That day, God gave me perspective. I need to focus on what I have, to be thankful for my son, and help him. That moment was pivotal.

The other crucial part of acceptance is educating yourself and others. It is exceptionally difficult to go it alone when raising a child on the autism spectrum. I will cover this further in the next chapter, but you need to find a core group that is willing to support you. This core group usually includes you as the parent(s), grandparents, siblings, aunts, uncles, cousins, and/or close friends. (I love the term *framily*—friends that are basically family.) Once you know who's on board and willing to do whatever it takes to assist your child, I suggest you encourage them to educate themselves on ASD, and you can help them do it.

After Gus was diagnosed, Michelle and I purchased the latest and best books and sent multiple copies to family members. From the very beginning, my father said to me, "Your mother and I want books and articles on autism. We want to immerse ourselves in the subject and learn everything we can." When your child is diagnosed with autism spectrum disorder, it is essential to have a core group of caring supporters by your side. After receiving the diagnosis, your close friends and family should have a rudimentary understanding of autism within two to three months. If they fail to take the initiative to research and understand your child's needs, then they may not be the right people for your core group.

You deserve people who genuinely care and make the effort to learn. Surrounding yourself with informed, compassionate allies is crucial. While it may seem harsh, this diagnosis is a defining moment—use it to distinguish who will stand with you and your child on this journey. With the right people in your corner, you will have the support and strength to navigate each day and each milestone ahead.

Nowadays, lack of education is inexcusable. (Since writing the book, I've re-immersed myself, and I am finding that there are so many wonderful new organizations, books, and resources that we did not have just a few years ago.) There are myriads of books, websites, and videos breaking down the basics of autism. If you and your core group are not doing your homework, ask yourself why not. There is no excuse not to become educated when it is so easy to do so.

Acceptance is multifaceted, and it leads to forward momentum. You are putting the car in drive and hitting the gas instead of remaining in neutral. Parenting a child on the spectrum takes a lot of effort, focus, and unrelenting love. You can't do it alone—you need many hands involved. Doing this by yourself will run you ragged. You have a choice: chaos versus focused love.

Chapter 3: It Takes a Village

"We rise by lifting others."[25]

– Robert G. Ingersoll

When Gus was diagnosed, we lived in a neighborhood with a lot of young, neurotypical boys who grew up together—many of whom were jocks. While most of the children in our neighborhood were running off to peewee football or little league, my son lacked motor skills and was in therapy.

As a parent of a child on the spectrum, you are not in the same social circles as other parents. The other parents got to know each other through common ground. They would meet up and trade stories about baseball tournaments and championship games, and we just couldn't relate. While those parents discussed weekends full of back-to-back ballgames, Michelle and I discussed the hours of therapy we had—there was no segue there. We were the outliers and felt alone.

Children with special needs tend to struggle with mainstream activities for a myriad of reasons, and Bob Brozovich, former North Fayette parks and recreation director, had a vision to help. Bob wanted full inclusion in the township, so he launched an email campaign asking if parents with special needs children wanted to start a group. The group would include children on the autism

---

[25] Robert G. Ingersoll. (n.d.). Goodreads. Retrieved December 27, 2023, from https://www.goodreads.com/quotes/8119455-we-rise-by-lifting-others

spectrum, Down syndrome, and children with cognitive or physical disabilities.

A dozen people immediately responded to Bob's email. My wife, Kelly Cain, Rebecca Lisotto, Linda Mullen, Diana Peligrino, Melissa Zirwas, Linda Mullen, and Debbie Unger were among the founding mothers in the organization. When searching for a name, member Ashleigh Smith brilliantly came up with PALS (Providing Assistance, Love & Support). I eventually joined the committee and became the voice for the organization. North Fayette PALS is "dedicated to developing and facilitating structured opportunities for children and youth with special needs in our community."[26] The organization offers participation in activities to build a community where citizens are treated with compassion and respect. The volunteer-run organization believes that all young people deserve a chance to shine. That is why they facilitate recreational activities that bring kids of all abilities together—these programs build bonds of compassion and respect between participants.

These types of communities and organizations are not only amazing for the children but also for meeting battle-tested parents whom you can relate to. Throughout the years, many of the original PALS families have become like family to us. Here, we met several parents with children who were roughly around the same level on the spectrum as Gus. Michelle and I found families that were in similar situations, and we quickly bonded. We finally found people who could relate to our experiences.

On a brief side note, Kelly Cain, one of the PALS founding mothers, launched The Autism Caring Center in 2017. I was honored to be one of the first individuals she asked to join her

---

[26] "Providing Assistance, Love & Support (PALS)," Township of North Fayette, https://north-fayette.com/202/Providing-Assistance-Love-Support-PALS.

board of directors. The "Autism Caring Center's mission is to enhance the lives of individuals and families by working diligently to provide support, resources, advocacy and offer training to community businesses to raise awareness and acceptance."[27] The center has become a beacon of light in the greater Pittsburgh area. It's a great example of how one person can make a significant difference. The center continues to grow and, to date, has assisted over 1,000 families. Kelly, as executive director of the center, has allowed me to greatly add to my village. Between North Fayette PALS and the Autism Caring Center, Kelly Cain and I have worked together, hand in hand, since 2010 to enhance the lives of special needs children.

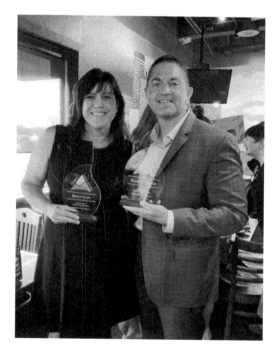

Kelly Cain and Me

[27] Autism Caring Center, https://autismcaringcenter.com/about-us.

It has been inspiring to meet countless loving and positive families that deal with circumstances similar to my own.

Having a child on the spectrum means a lot of isolation. When you first get the diagnosis, it can feel like you are the only person on the planet experiencing what you are going through. First, exhale. You are *not* the only one going through this, I promise you that. I know it is not easy, but there are other people going through this, too. You just need to find them and start building a village—a village of support, a village of love, a village of empathy. The autism community is vast, loving, experienced, and willing to help.

Now more than ever, there are communities, organizations, and activities where kids on the spectrum can get together and do things. When you are in amongst that mix, you meet battle-tested parents in a similar situation. You find people who can act as a sounding board to exchange ideas with. Maybe they can even introduce you to new modalities. At the very least, you might find an empathetic ear to listen and offer assurance that you are not in this alone. You might be thinking, *But Harry, what if I conduct a thorough search online and cannot seem to find a local support group or organization in my area?* My suggestion: *Be a difference maker and create one.*

I tell both of my sons on a regular basis, "In life, you have two options: sit on the bench or play in the game. The people who play in the game make the difference." According to the CDC (Centers for Disease Control and Prevention), one in 36 children are now diagnosed with autism.[28] Just a few years ago the statistic was one in 44. There is a very high probability that other families in your area have children on the spectrum. Instead of finding your village, you can build one.

---

[28]"Autism Spectrum Disorder (ASD)," Centers for Disease Control and Prevention, https://www.cdc.gov/ncbddd/autism/data.html.

Regardless of a couple's determination to love their child or children on the spectrum, the diagnosis of ASD immediately adds complexity to their lives. This is an exceptionally difficult time for any couple. I cannot stress enough that after diagnosis, and acceptance, you need to gather a team of support. This starts with your family. Close friends you consider family, better known as *framily*, fall into this category as well. Remember to remain patient throughout this process. Friends and family are digesting the new normal and dealing with their own emotions. The last thing anyone needs is ridicule or negativity. Clear lines of communication are critical. Do not be afraid to let them know what you need. Those needs will range from emotional (a hug, support, love) to material (financial assistance, food, rides).

Michelle and I are fortunate. We were quick to receive a tidal wave of love and support from our friends and family. They repeatedly asked us, "What can we do to help?"

My older brother, Michael, has always been a hero to me, and especially during this journey. The moment he heard about Gus's diagnosis, Michael stepped up without hesitation. He became my impromptu psychologist, lending an ear during my hardest days. Together with my sister-in-law, Robin, they were remarkably supportive. They'd call just to check on Gus's progress and our wellbeing. Aware of the steep costs that came with supporting a child on the spectrum, their generosity knew no bounds. "Let us take care of that," they would often say. Even when we refused their help, it didn't matter. Within a day, a check would arrive in the mail. We are so grateful for their kindness and generosity. Without their support, there are treatments we never could have tried. They went above and beyond to help us give Gus every possible chance. We will never forget what they did for us ... for Gus.

Michelle and I were fortunate to have the majority of our family focused on one goal: making Gus the best that he could be. I could go on, but I have a finite number of words I can write in this book. I cannot express the appreciation I have for my family and the supportive and nurturing environment they created for my son.

My parents were superhuman in their support throughout Gus's journey. I cannot say enough about them. They were willing, at any point, to take us anywhere, anytime—whether to therapy or to give Michelle and me a needed a break and a chance to be together as a couple. Sometimes, while we were away in therapy, my parents would show up at our house with food and coffee ready for us when we returned. If Michelle or I were ill, or unable to drive Gus, we could always count on *Papou* and *Yia Yia*. The "taxi" was readily available. Every therapist and teacher who ever worked with Gus became best friends with *Papou* and *Yia Yia*. To this day, when Michelle and I run into one of Gus's past therapists or teachers, they immediately ask, "How are your parents? We really miss them." It is truly hard to articulate the level of love, support, patience, and devotion they displayed throughout Gus's many, many hours of therapy.

English scholar, librarian, biographer, and poet, Richard Garnett, once stated, "Love is the greatest gift one generation can leave another."[29] My parents have delivered this gift in spades for both of my sons. I would be remiss if I did not highlight the special bond between my father and Gus. They were inseparable, and I would refer to them as the "dynamic duo." My father took Gus everywhere—local malls, parks, restaurants, activities, therapy. There were local restaurants that knew them so well that they would immediately submit their order when my father pulled up to the restaurant. They achieved celebrity status!

---

[29] "The Most Beautiful Grandparents Day Quotes," Hooray Heros, https://hoorayheroes.com/stories/the-most-beautiful-grandparents-day-quotes/.

He was with us at Cleveland Clinic when Gus was officially diagnosed with autism and was heavily involved in school and therapy well into his teen years. Gus was *everything* to my father and watching Gus succeed became his obsession.

It was an atomic bomb of devastation to our family when my father passed away in June of 2023 after valiantly fighting stage IV lung cancer and a stroke. Minutes before closing his casket, my brilliant brother, Michael—in an act of sheer class, selflessness, and love—brought Gus over to the casket. My brother looked at Gus and said, "You were his alpha and his omega." Although Michael is immensely generous and has given me many gifts in my life, none will ever surpass that moment. (May my father's memory be eternal.)

I am cognizant there are families that may be on their own. However, if you do not have a support system of family or close friends, then I would encourage you to find a community that you can relate to. Even if you do not have one at the moment, you have to look for or create one.

Not sure where to start? Look for local groups through social media or outlets like the Autism Caring Center. Google autism conferences near you, and attend, but do not go to the conference and sit alone in a corner. Spend time speaking with other moms and dads while you are there. Gather phone numbers and connect on social platforms.

You cannot be a lone wolf in this situation; you just cannot be. There is so much time involved between running to therapy and the doctor's office and socializing—you need to have people there who have your back. Do not attempt to be a stand-alone superhero. Children, regardless of where they are on the spectrum, improve with collective love. Just keep rowing that boat forward, and good things will happen.

Chapter 4: The Mind of a Black Belt: The 2% Rule

"Make at least one definite move daily toward your goal."[30]

– Bruce Lee

Anyone taking any form of martial arts starts at a novice, or a white belt level. As the New Zealand Disability Karate Association so eloquently puts it, "The white belt is the beginning of life's cycle and represents the seed as it lies beneath the snow in winter."[31] To proceed to the next belt color, the student must practice daily to become proficient in a series of forms, blocks, punches, and kicks.

I have a background in Tang Soo Do, and we would start every class with the same fundamental strikes—same punches, same kicks. For some, the redundancy might be maddening. (Anyone watching us would think we were out of our minds.) However, there is a reason for this methodology. Bruce Lee once stated, "I fear not the man who has practiced 10,000 kicks once, but I fear the man who has practiced one kick 10,000 times."[32]

---

[30] Great Bruce Lee Quotes | Sources of Insight. https://sourcesofinsight.com/bruce-lee-quotes/

[31] "Our Mission," New Zealand Disability Karate Association, https://www.karatedojo.nz/cgi-bin/nzdkaMission.cgi#:~:text=The%20white%20belt%20is%20the.
[32] Devon Boorman, "Bruce Lee's 10,000 Kicks and the Real Meaning of Mastery," Academie Duello(blog),

The goal here is incremental improvement, each and every class. You are developing muscle memory. You do not even think about it or realize how much better you are getting.

White belts may start by throwing a beginner punch, thrusting their first forward without moving their body or rotating their hand. Whereas, the black belt, after throwing thousands upon thousands of punches, knows "no hips, no punch." They understand that the power comes from your feet and your hips. They're twisting their hips with the full weight of their body and striking with the correct protruding knuckles.

When you get to the black belt level, everything is synaptically connected, and you flow—but to get there is an evolution. Every black belt is a white belt that never refused to quit.

The same concept applies to parents with a child on the autism spectrum. If you are willing to show the determination of a black belt, small incremental wins will lead to sizable gains. This is what I call the 2% rule, and it is something I preach about every day. My 2% rule is an extension of my experience with martial arts. It takes an exceptional amount of determination, sacrifice, and the same level of patience while working with your child every day to make subtle improvements.

James Clear developed a similar mindset in his New York Times bestseller, Atomic Habits. Clear defines atomic habits as being small habits that are part of a bigger system of changing your life with self-awareness, goal setting, and actions.[33]

---

https://www.academieduello.com/news-blog/bruce-lees-1000-kicks-and-the-real-meaning-of-mastery/
[33] Atomic Habits by James Clear: Book Summary and Insights (calvinrosser.com). https://calvinrosser.com/notes/atomic-

Entering your day with the 2% mindset when working with your child is like establishing atomic habits for improvement. These tiny wins lead to large victories. You have to have an outlook that believes small wins on a daily basis will lead to sizable wins in the future. I want parents to wake up every day and state, "I want to make my child 2% better at (fill in the blank)."

What do these improvements look like? It will vary greatly per child. Children with ASD are unique and can be vastly different from one another. The improvement could be anything from listening to speaking, fine motor skills work, activities of daily living, homework, feeding themselves, or trying a new food texture. Michelle and I would go into each day looking for something Gus could improve 2% on, whether it was behaviorally, educationally, or daily living activities.

When Gus was young, he was obsessed with fans. I was never shy about taking either of my sons out shopping with me, but trips to Home Depot and Lowe's could be taxing. If Gus was within eyesight of the fan department, he would insist on staying there for a long time. The entire department captivated him. He would wander up and down the aisle, staring up at the whirling blades, his neck swiveling slowly to match their rhythmic rotation. I would sometimes look at him helplessly, wishing I could enter Gus's world, if only for a moment, to understand what brought him such fascination and peace. Eventually my patience would grow thin, and frustrated, I would finally say, "Enough Gus! We're leaving," and he would break down crying.

I would often have to pick him up, screaming and flailing, and carry him out of the store. As we caused a scene, I could feel the eyes of other customers on us, judging me, and likely thinking,

---

habits/#:~:text=An%20atomic%20habit%20is%20a,changes%20to%20create%20remarkable%20results.

What a terrible father. It was painful and isolating, but Gus couldn't help it—the lights, sounds, and overstimulation of the store could send him into sensory overload. As many of you reading this book know, as a parent of an autistic child, I learned to grow thick skin and have compassion for what my child was experiencing.

The road to overcoming obsession was long and winding for Gus. Day after day, month after month, we trudged through ABA therapy, slowly untangling his fixations on fans, hinges, and more. It was a marathon, not a sprint—a journey marked by tiny steps forward (2% steps) and the occasional backslide.

One year later we ventured into our local Home Depot. I grabbed a few items then took him by the fan department.

I told him, "I will let you look at the fans for ten minutes then we have to leave."

He quickly stated, "OK, Dad."

The minutes crawled by as I stood watching him, the anticipation building inside me. Ten minutes felt more like an eternity as I waited for the precious time to end.

Finally, I bent down and said, "OK, buddy, time is up. We have to go now."

He looked at me with his big eyes, calm and serene, and replied, "OK, Dad, we can go."

No kicking, no screaming, no crying—just simple acceptance. Remember, the 2% rule is about small, incremental wins that lead to sizable victories. That day in Home Depot was the definition of a sizable victory.

I want to emphasize that we love every bit of Gus, every bit of his DNA. At the end of the day, you must remember that you are not trying to change the actual human being that they are. Will you get to a point where you feel discouraged working toward those improvements? Yes, but the feeling of being discouraged simply means you are human, and I think we need to recognize that. As Frederick Douglass once said, "If there is no struggle, there is no progress."[34]

It is human nature to get upset, to get depressed, to feel that frustration. When Gus was going through all the therapies as a child, we were told verbatim that we had *normalized* Gus. (You do not hear that often in the struggle with a child on the spectrum.) Then he put on those damn Crocs, fell down the steps, and lost everything. If you do not think I cried, I did. It is human to have those feelings, but you need to stay the course. It is OK to give yourself a day to lean into those feelings, but you need to change that quickly—you need to do it for your child.

Motivational speaker Dr. Eric Thomas has a quote that has always stuck with me, "Recycle your pain, allow your pain to reach you to greatness."[35] At the time that Gus fell, we were delivered quite a blow. From a fighting standpoint, we were on guard, getting hit: ground and pound. After the initial shock, I sat there, did some deep breathing, and then said, "It is time to fight back. There is no other option for this kid. I am going to keep moving forward, churning the boat, get everybody's spirits up, and keep going."

---

[34] Frederick Douglass, (1857) "If There Is No Struggle, There Is No Progress" • (blackpast.org). https://www.blackpast.org/african-american-history/1857-frederick-douglass-if-there-no-struggle-there-no-progress/
[35] Eric Thomas Quotes That Will Motivate You to Dream More. (2020, January 9). https://motivation2life.com/motivational-quotes-from-eric-thomas/.

We lost years of therapy when Gus fell, but, ultimately, love and toughness prevailed, and he progressed. He wouldn't be in college right now if we had not continued to fight for him. I do not know where he would be. You just have to stay the course, fight the fight, and keep moving forward. Remember, you are the captain of the ship, and your job is to keep sailing.

As the parent of a child with mild autism, I have had many conversations with parents of children that are moderate to severe on the spectrum. They have approached me at fundraisers and speaking engagements and often ask me how their child can make daily progress. Many indicated they did not think it was possible.

I understand the frustration and hopelessness that can set in when progress seems slow, but I urge you—do not give up hope. Your child's wins may not look like what you expected, but they are still wins. A new way of communicating through sign language or picture cards is an incredible achievement. Mastering activities of daily living that once seemed impossible is a major victory. Will a child with severe autism's win look differently from my son's? Absolutely, but a win is a win. Progress is progress.

To quote former Georgetown Hoya and Miami Heat star, Alonzo Mourning, "A win is a win, regardless of how you look at it."[36] You can achieve the 2% improvement with any child on the spectrum. I truly believe that. Focus on incremental improvement. Celebrate the small wins, even if they look different than the milestones other children reach, meet them where they are, acknowledge their challenges, and help them feel empowered by praising each tiny step forward. With an emphasis on patience and

---

[36] Alonzo Mourning Quote: "A win is a win, regardless of how you look at it." (n.d.). Quotefancy.com. Retrieved December 27, 2023, from https://quotefancy.com/quote/1336000/Alonzo-Mourning-A-win-is-a-win-regardless-of-how-you-look-at-it#:~:text=Alonzo%20Mourning%20Quote%3A%20.

compassionate support and a commitment to steady (if slow) progress, their growth will come.

You need to go into the 2% rule with the understanding that you are not going to change things overnight. Choose one activity at a time and attempt to improve it by 2%. Seismic changes are tough to come by, but incremental improvements are the key, and they add up over time. You want collective wins, not a grand slam. If you stick with the idea that this is a marathon, not a sprint, you will keep yourself sane.

Chapter 5: Do Not Forget to Smile

"Self-care is giving the world the best of you, instead of what's left of you."[37]

– Katie Reed

There will be times when you experience feelings of exhaustion and frustration or even bouts of depression when you are parenting a child on the spectrum. When you are in the early stages, you are navigating unchartered territory. If one parent is having a bad day at work and comes home to the child melting down, it can be a recipe for disaster.

In the thick of the chaos, I want you to try something. First, separate yourself from the situation. Then, go into another room to give yourself some quiet time … and smile. *Smile? Seriously? Seriously.*

The human body is incredible, and a smile is powerful. Think of it as a signal that activates a change of mindset. You know when you have a tech issue, the first thing you are asked to do is reset the device? It is the same idea. A smile forces a reset in the brain, and there is science behind this. Believe it or not, even a brief smile releases tiny molecules, called neuropeptides, that help fight off stress.[38] You are essentially telling your body that, regardless of the

---

[37] Perfect Self-Care Quotes to Nurture Your Mental Health - The Woods At Parkside. (2020, January 2). Www.thewoodsatparkside.com. https://www.thewoodsatparkside.com/7-perfect-self-care-quotes-to-nurture-your-mental-health/

[38] Graham, A. (n.d.). When the well runs dry: A personal hygiene

shitty situation, you are happy. When you smile brightly, it activates neurotransmitters in the body and calms it down. Dopamine, serotonin, and endorphins come into play as well. Without getting too technical, dopamine is what gives you feelings of pleasure and motivation, endorphins are pain relievers, and serotonin is an antidepressant.[39] All of this is triggered by a 30-second smile? *Yes.* (Incredible, huh?)

Smiling is a quick and easy coping technique—think of it as two minutes of mental yoga. This can also be accompanied by a mantra. Remember the commonly used phrase, "this too shall pass"? No matter how bad of a day you are having, *this too shall pass.* Do not wait until you are in the midst of having a horrific day or moment to try out the smile rule. Start now.

Before you even get out of bed each morning, I want you to lock in your day with an ear-to-ear smile. Your spouse may think you have a stash of cannabis or magic mushrooms that you got into, but do not worry about what someone else may think of you. After you smile, focus on breathing. I prefer a popular technique known as "box breathing," which refers to the fact that a box has four sides. It's also known as Sama Vritti Pranayama[40] from the yoga practice known as "pranayama." Box breathing can lower your blood pressure and immediately provide a sense of calm. Breathe in for four seconds slowly. Allow your brain to feel the air flow into your

---

discussion. The Courier-Journal. Retrieved January 17, 2024, from https://eu.courier-journal.com/story/life/2022/03/11/when-well-runs-dry-personal-hygiene-discussion/9448528002/

[39] Mark Stibich, PhD, 10 Big Benefits of Smiling (verywellmind.com) (verywellmind.com).
[40] Timothy Burgin. (2021, June 8). Sama Vritti Pranayama (Box Breath or Equal Breathing) • Yoga Basics. Yoga Basics. https://www.yogabasics.com/practice/sama-vritti-pranayama/#:~:text=Sama%20Vritti%20Pranayama%20is%20a

lungs. Hold the breath for four seconds; then slowly exhale through your mouth for four seconds, hold your breath again for four more seconds.

You can repeat these steps until you feel centered. You may be wondering why I am talking about the science of a smile and box breathing when you are here looking for ideas to parent your autistic child. Parents with a child or children on the spectrum deal with a myriad of issues: meltdowns, rigidities, oppositional defiance, irritability, communication challenges, financial stress, and stigmatization. You need to have go-to techniques to lower your stress. We know that a consistent amount of stress can be debilitating on the mind and body. This is why I want you to be the optimal version of yourself every day as you parent your child.

People tend to forget the root cause of experiencing stress stems from caring deeply about something. The stress I experienced was often when I wanted Gus to do his best, and we encountered a setback. It was the internal pain of knowing that we hit a speed bump or lost ground in our efforts to help him. Maybe you can relate.

When I experienced these moments of stress and frustration, I found myself gravitating to an isolated spot in my house or elsewhere, smiling, breathing, and attempting to change my mindset. If you feel stressed or overwhelmed, try to find a quiet space, and reset. I prefer a parent that is stressed because they care over one who is apathetic or non-existent in their child's life, but you must keep your stress in check.

Your child is counting on you—always keep that in mind. You have to remember you are the captain of the ship. If you are in a state of chaos, your family and your children will be in a state of chaos. Yes, your stress will permeate a household, and nothing good comes from that. And if you have a behavior specialist or trained staff support person working with your child in your home, you have just added to their stress as well. Stress and negative energy are toxic. Learn to take a minute, reset your brain, and tackle the day with a calm and positive mindset.

Will you inevitably feel irritated, fly off the handle, swear, or yell at your spouse, or child? Yes, you are human. Will a smile be enough for those moments? Maybe not, but it is a temporary reprieve. In a short period of time, you are forcing the endorphins to show up and remind you, *This too shall pass. I need to calm down and set the example. I need to be strong and the pillar of the family.* A smile is a 30-second cheat code to change your mindset, and box breathing is comparable to hitting a systemic pressure valve. If the days get totally overwhelming, and you have someone to help at home, find a stress reliever away from your house. My preferred release is going to the gym and hitting the heavy bag. (I have always been a boxer, having that fighter mentality.) When I was pounding the bag, I could feel my frustrations being expunged from my body. I felt far better when I was done. For you, the release may be yoga or meditation. Because that might not always be feasible, a smile or breathing can fill the gaps.

That said, setting aside time to be active whenever possible and releasing frustrations is not optional; it is a necessity. The better shape you are in, the better you can tackle this long journey with your child. If you are head of the household, Dad, you need to set the example. You should strive to be in great shape mentally *and* physically.

This isn't meant to be an exercise book but let me share a quote from human potential thought leader, Bryant McGill, "Taking care of yourself is the most powerful way to begin to take care of others."

[41] This brilliant quote comes from his book, *Simple Reminders: Inspiration for Living Your Best Life*. I emphatically agree with this statement. Parents with children on the autism spectrum have an exceptionally rigorous schedule: the daily role of parenting, individualized education program (IEP) meetings, therapy, physician visits, monitoring and adhering to a specialized diet, a unique supplementation schedule ... the list is endless. (Oh, and you still may have neurotypical siblings to parent!) The Bottom line is you are the leader of your child's overall development, and that requires optimal health and energy.

If you are sitting on the couch consuming fast food, processed junk, and rarely moving, you are setting a bad example for your child. Not only that, but you'll lack the daily energy needed to keep up with the demands of being a special needs parent.

Your body is a machine. It will run at peak performance if you consume the proper fuel. I usually do not consume food I cannot find in the forest or the sea. You will not find donuts, Doritos, or potato chips out in nature. Do not get me wrong, if my sons have a birthday party, yes, I will have a piece of cake. (I am not that draconian with what I eat.)

However, I immediately go back to eating healthy, organic, grass-fed foods. Limit your intake of refined carbohydrates, sugar (the ultimate devil), and seed oils. Forget the word "diet"; a diet is a con job. Diets are temporary and futile. What you want to do is create a healthy lifestyle.

Eating cleaner, healthier food sets a great example for your children. You can encourage them to replicate your eating, even if

---

[41] McGill, B., & McGill, J. Y. Simple Reminders: Inspiration for Living Your Best Life (Kindle Edition) [Review of Simple Reminders: Inspiration for Living Your Best Life]. SRN Publishing. (2018).

you substitute one item at a time. Single ingredient foods—foods that have only themselves listed in the ingredient lines—like carrots, apples, pears, bananas are phenomenal substitutions for junk and processed foods.

To quote the brilliant author Michael Pollan, "Real food grows, rots, dies. Real food doesn't need an ingredient label. Real food doesn't make claims."[42] You know it is healthy. Processed, sugar-laden foods alter your child neurologically.

I am cognizant that fast food is inexpensive, but it contains excessive amounts of sugar, saturated and/or trans fats, processed preservatives, and other ingredients. (There is no way you will feel good or be at your best if you are constantly consuming those.) If you want your child 2% better, find clean organic ingredients. Food dyes are detrimental as well. Studies have shown food dyes pose health risks ranging from hyperactivity to ADHD and cancer.[43] Fascinating research has emerged on the connections between nutrition and autism spectrum disorder. Studies have also shown that certain dietary interventions may help improve symptoms and overall wellbeing for children on the spectrum.[44] The brain is intricately linked to the gut, and the food we eat provides the building blocks for brain development and function. Some researchers hypothesize that inflammation, immune system

---

[42] Michael Pollan, *Food Rules: An Eater's Manual*, (New York, Penguin Press), 2011.

[43] "Food Dyes: A Rainbow of Risk," Center for Science in the Public Interest, https://www.cspinet.org/resource/food-dyes-rainbow-risks.

[44] Doreswamy S, Bashir A, Guarecuco J E, et al. (December 22, 2020) Effects of Diet, Nutrition, and Exercise in Children With Autism and Autism Spectrum Disorder: A Literature Review. Cureus 12(12): e12222. doi:10.7759/cureus.12222, https://doi.org/10.7759/cureus.12222.

abnormalities, oxidative stress, and gut microbiome imbalances may underlie autism's core symptoms. Strategies like eliminating gluten and casein, adding probiotics and omega-3s, and removing processed foods have shown promise in reducing gastrointestinal issues, boosting focus and attention, decreasing repetitive behaviors, and improving communication and social skills for children on the spectrum.

More research is needed in this area, but it is clear that diet can impact the vulnerable autistic brain. There is hope that continued work in this exciting area may uncover targeted nutritional therapies for improving brain connectivity and future outcomes in autism.

I realize I sound like I am preaching, but this is far from a new concept. Hippocrates, the father of modern medicine and fellow Greek (*OPA!*), stated, "Let food be thy medicine and medicine be thy food."[45] Improving your diet is the first major step when it comes to self-care. Replicating healthy eating with your child is the logical next step.

The 2% rule also applies to improving your child's health. It is far from an overnight process but well worth the effort. Remember the "beige diet" our sons were obsessed with? (I am sure many of you can relate.) It consisted of *nothing* but exotic items like chicken nuggets, French fries, and white bread. The elimination of gluten and casein, and implementation of healthier food was a slow and arduous process. With time, patience, and unrelenting love, you can accomplish the task. Your child will feel better, act better, and have sharper mental acuity.

---

[45] Richard Smith (Editor), "Let food be thy medicine ...," National Library of Medicine, BMJ. 2004 Jan 24; 328(7433): 0., https://www.ncbi.nlm.nih.gov/pmc/articles/PMC318470/.

Self-care applies equally to parents and children. Movement is a critical part of that and essential for all bodies. I have already mentioned modeling healthy eating habits, now I want to discuss the importance of physical activity, especially for children with autism. The benefits of exercise are far-reaching. It can enhance physical and mental health in profound ways, but the question remains: How do you motivate a child who prefers solo, sedentary activities with creativity and compassion?

Many children with autism would rather play video games than run around outside. Consequently, studies show nearly half of these children are overweight or obese, elevating their risk for diabetes and hypertension.[46] This is alarming, yet surmountable. With your encouragement, physical activity can become a rewarding part of their routine. Patience and imagination may be required, but you can find activities your child truly enjoys. The key is making exercise social and interactive. You can invite friends or siblings to play tag or kick a ball, explore community sports teams tailored to children with special needs, or lead family bike rides and/or hikes in nature. Let your child's interests guide you. Move together in ways that spark their passion and bring them joy.

There are numerous sports and activities tailored for children with ASD: golf, martial arts, bowling, running, horseback riding, swimming, dance, yoga, biking, tennis, and skiing. The possibilities are endless. Physical activity is vital for your child's health and wellbeing, and with creativity and compassion you can make exercise fun.

---

[46] Brandy E. Strahan and Jennifer H. Elder, "Video Game Playing Effects on Obesity in an Adolescent with Autism Spectrum Disorder: A Case Study," Hindawi, Volume 2015 | Article ID 128365 | https://doi.org/10.1155/2015/128365.

Gus struggled with organized sports, but he was able to achieve a red belt in Tang Soo Do, run several 5K races, and he loves to mountain bike. Stay positive, creative, and consistent. Help your child discover the power and pleasure of an active body. Their increased health and happiness will be all the thanks you need.

I can already hear some of you saying, *Harry, you just listed a grueling schedule, how am I supposed to find time for self-care, like eating healthy and exercising?* I embody former United States Navy Seal, author, and motivational speaker, David Goggins's *no bullshit, no excuses mentality.* I do not "preach" anything I do not practice myself, so my answer? Make the time to get off your ass and move! *No excuses.* Whether it is one hour or squeezing in 15 minutes, a little movement is better than none. Michelle and I would often take turns watching our sons to allow the other to have an hour to move. I often preferred running, martial arts, lifting weights, or hitting the heavy bag. It was a catharsis. The gym, dojo, or nature trail became a sanctuary for me to release my tension, ramp up my energy levels, and keep myself in optimal shape for my sons, my wife, and our shared mission to make Gus the best that he could be. Self-care is critical for parents who have children on the spectrum. You'll feel better, look better, have more energy, and set a great example for your children. Parents of ASD children should train like warriors because it's a long (and often grueling) journey.

Chapter 6: Keeping Your Eyes on the Prize: Having Sight and Vision

"The only thing worse than being blind is having sight but not vision."[47]

– Helen Keller

If you have a goal without a destination in mind, you will not have a clear path for achieving it. Goals are only meaningful when they are tied to a vision. Imagine you want to travel to Europe one day, but do not know what documentation you'll need or modes of transportation you need to get there. That will make for a difficult trip. Vision provides you with a clear path to achievement.

As a parent, you must have vision, but you also need sight. What is the difference? Vision is looking toward the future, whereas sight is focusing on the present; it is mindfulness. It is shutting everything else down and focusing on what's in the now. You have to look at the context of what's going on presently with your child to help inform the future. A parent of a neurotypical child can usually focus on the now without the same intensity of worry about the future as a parent of a special needs child, but a parent with a child on the spectrum *always* has to think of both.

To break these down even further, sight involves the 2% rule. It means focusing on making those every day slight improvements. The way to keep your sight (the *now* goals) in check is by having a

---

47 Campaign 1. (n.d.). Roger Osbaldiston. Retrieved December 19, 2023, from https://rogerosbaldiston.com/passionvisionaction

vision for your child's future. Vision is thinking about where your child is now and how to get him or her where you want in five years, ten years.

I know it is easy to get caught in the day-to-day grind, especially in those early years. You might have people at your house for therapy, sunup to sundown, and assignments to work on with your child in between. You are on call 24/7, so it can be easy to fall into the sight aspect and completely forget about the vision piece, but you must keep both in mind. You cannot steer a car unless you grip the wheel, right? Keeping an eye on that long-term vision is what's going to help you stay focused now.

Your vision for your child may change depending upon where he or she is now. If you go to a PALS event, you'll see children who range from mild or moderate to severe. The vision for each child will look different and is subject to change depending on the child's progress. Remember to focus on 2% daily improvements to get to your vision. For a family with a severely autistic child who is unable to speak, the vision might be getting him or her to talk. Therapy might be the sight part of the equation. They are probably trying everything possible to help their child right now to make daily improvements (however slight) while keeping an eye on the distant prize.

If the child remains unable to speak, they may have to reevaluate their vision. Perhaps that means getting the child an assisted technology device for communication. (Children have voices; sometimes they need to be electronic.) Another example would be an adult who is severely autistic, still living at home, and completely unable to take care of himself or herself independently. The vision will look very different for this individual. It might include looking into home health options or determining who will be the primary caretaker.

For Michelle and me, our vision for Gus was college and maturation. When he was in middle school, we did not know if Gus would make it to college. Still, that was our vision. When Gus hit high school, after the Brain Balance years, I had more confidence that we could get him to college. Michelle and I attempted to do everything we could to prepare Gus through high school, focusing on the 2% rule. Things were not perfect, but he was thriving. Gus had his posse of friends and a 3.8 GPA.

We have achieved the vision we set for Gus; he successfully transitioned to college and is currently in school. This next stage of life has presented new challenges, and we need to reevaluate both our sight and vision. Social connections are difficult, and Gus struggles with preparation for exams. His grades are passable but less than stellar. It is tempting to get caught up in worries of failure or about him dropping out, but Michelle and I choose to refocus our sight.

What can we do *now* to help him? College is a time for growth, and with continued guidance, we know Gus can find his footing. He is doing everything right—attending class, taking diligent notes, and listening actively to his professors. The one missing piece is mastering the art of test-taking. With guidance to develop effective study and test-taking strategies, Gus can unlock his full potential on exams. Helping him gain these skills now will equip Gus with the tools to excel throughout his remaining three years of college. Mastering this critical skill set, he can fully leverage his responsible work ethic and transform his academic experience.

We gathered to develop a strategy for success, a true battle plan. Kent State offers courses on how to sharpen study skills and improve test taking. Gus scheduled a number of them. To stay connected, he chose to regularly check in with his professors. I lined up tutors, conveniently located near campus for extra help in difficult classes. Gus spoke with Kent State's student accessibility services (SAS), and they offer a number of services to assist him in the classroom. He has been doing everything we asked of him; we simply needed to bridge the gap. (If he was not attending class and was totally isolated, I would have been concerned.) Our battle plan is paying off, and Gus is starting to make strides in the classroom. If we have to refocus our sight again, we will do so. Our vision for our son right now is finishing his degree, possibly getting a second. I am hoping the vision stays there, but if the struggle continues, we might have to adjust our vision. Gus understands the value of an education and is doing everything it takes to obtain his degree. We remain focused on getting him in a position where he is making money, able to live on his own, and have a happy life.

I mentioned Gus has been struggling to find his social footing. (Yes, we have a sight plan for that as well.) Kent State boasts an impressive 300+ clubs, and he plans to sign up for a few of them and connect with peers who have shared interests. On top of club involvement, he is excited to rush a fraternity and find his community. We were lucky enough to discover a personal trainer at Kent State who Gus really clicks with. He will be training with him at least three times a week, which is not only great for his health but also represents another chance to cultivate meaningful relationships. With the rich social landscape at Kent State and Gus's eagerness to put himself out there, I am confident he will find fulfilling friendships and continue to flourish.

As parents, we get lost in the details of each day, trying to navigate the unpredictable waters of autism. But we must keep our eyes fixed on the horizon, on the vision we hold for our children's future. Though every child's path is unique, our hopes remain the same: to see him or her thrive and find joy. When breakthroughs come, we rejoice, knowing our vision is within reach. Each new therapy or new medicine that unlocks their potential brings our dreams closer. The vision shifts and comes into sharper focus.

My prayer for you, dear parent, is that your vision becomes reality; that you will watch your child grow and blossom in ways you once only dreamed of. Stay anchored to that vision, as we have done, even when the way is hard. Breakthrough by breakthrough, we will get there. Our children will flourish, and our boldest hopes will be fulfilled.

Chapter 7: Finding Your Max and Your Jakub

"Loyalty is when you have my back behind my back."[48]

– Matt Tolbert

Even though I am the vice president of my church, I have a very quiet, convicting faith. I won't bombard you with scripture quotes or preach at you to convert. I don't cloister myself away in a strictly Christian world of music and movies. I enjoy listening to heavy metal and punk rock, and I watch R-rated movies, but make no mistake, I live what I believe. As I often say, "If you are breathing air, you should be helping others." My faith in God runs deep, even if I don't shout it from the rooftops. I aim to reflect my beliefs through my daily actions.

I believe God does everything for a reason, and so I believe He handed you your child exactly the way he or she is supposed to be. In some ways, I think God handed me—and you—a child who needs some extra work because He believes in us.

Our children were given to us *as is*, so we should appreciate their extraordinary gifts, strengths, and what it is they bring to the world. My two sons are wildly different. Gus is our happy hippie. He is gentle, sweet, and always beaming with positivity and a smile. Max, his younger brother, is an edgy, competitive athlete. He

---

[48] Matt Tolbert, "I Got Your Back Quotes to Help You Remember You Are Not Alone," Everyday Power, https://everydaypower.com/i-got-your-back-quotes/.

committed to playing football for Allegheny College in Meadville, Pa. (Go Gators!) Max has a heart of gold but is far different than Gus. Despite their differences, Max has always deeply admired Gus and always has his back. Over time, Max started to realize Gus was a bit different. Not a lot, Gus is mild on the spectrum, but we still had to have *that* discussion.

When it came time to explain to Max that his brother's brain functions differently than ours, and he has autistic traits, I used an analogy—one that I'd recommend to any parent of a child on the spectrum to start a dialogue with siblings: "You and I, our brains are a PC. Your [brother or sister] is an Apple. They might function and process a little bit differently, but ultimately, we are all the same."

Our brains are computers, right? So, I always recommend explaining it this way.

Siblings are invaluable companions on an autistic child's journey. They are more than playmates: they are guides into the social world. With patience and compassion, brothers and sisters can gently coax their autistic sibling into new experiences and model age-appropriate behavior. Laughter, empathy, and carefree fun with a neurotypical sibling provides an autistic child acceptance and understanding they may struggle to find elsewhere. Though the role is often thrust upon them unexpectedly, siblings can rise to meet the needs of their autistic brother or sister. Their support and friendship impart confidence and skills that last a lifetime. For children with autism, the unbreakable bond with a sibling is a lifeline to connect with the world around them.

A sibling bond is like no other. Growing up with an autistic brother or sister is a profound experience that shapes them in unforgettable ways. Though the journey is filled with challenges, the rewards are just as abundant. Autistic siblings teach patience and compassion from a young age. They show us a different perspective of the world that is often more imaginative and insightful. We become more attuned to others' needs and learn to communicate in creative ways. There is great joy in celebrating the smallest of milestones. This special relationship brings out an inner strength and resilience.

They gain wisdom beyond their years. The empathy and advocacy skills that are developed ripple out, inspiring them to stand up for others. Better yet, their capacity for unconditional love expands. Yes, there are hard days when they feel the weight of responsibility on their young shoulders, but there is also laughter and silliness. There are hugs and inside jokes. There is pride in seeing their sibling thrive.

Growing up together, they are bonded for life. Autistic siblings profoundly shape their brothers and sisters to be more compassionate, patient, and caring human beings. They are forever changed and likely forever grateful.

My other recommendation to parents is to give your neurotypical child, or children, as much time and love as their sibling(s) on the spectrum. I would also encourage any neurotypical siblings to get as involved as possible. Let them know that they are a critical part of the team, that they can be of great assistance to their sibling, and then define what you mean by *assistance*. If there is a child who is moderate to severe, it takes a different level of understanding. Assistance may look like that sibling helping with activities of daily living. In other words, that sibling becomes an extension of the parents in helping their brother or sister get better with their day-to-day tasks.

This could be encouraging their brother or sister to try new foods or working with them to settle after a meltdown. I understand that having a child help calm his or her sibling down when they are having a meltdown is a different level—but that does not mean they should not be involved. Asking them to participate in the care of their neurodivergent sibling can and should be done. It is a tougher ask when you get into the moderate to severe range for a sibling, and it takes a special kid to do that. But neurotypical siblings can really help in this journey for improvement, regardless of where your child is on the spectrum.

In our family, Max's assistance with Gus meant in a social context. Gus is mild on the spectrum and lived a somewhat typical teenage life. For instance, he grappled with social issues, like social media. As the maturation of both our sons kicked in, Max stepped in to help Gus in every way he could. If Max noticed Gus was in an awkward social interaction, he would always recommend how Gus could do something differently. Max would correct Gus's social media posts to help make them "cool," and would evaluate outfits his brother wore. Max was perpetually swagged out in the latest fashions. (I say Max has fashion tastes somewhere between a pimp and Elton John—real attention getters!) Max was always there to help Gus out if he needed a correction, especially with the color coordination of his wardrobe.

There were times when Gus would confound Max with a certain behavior, and it would inevitably lead to an argument. Michelle and I would acknowledge their feelings and discuss their behavior and reactions to the behavior. Finding a palpable, mutually agreed upon solution to the flare up would inevitably lead to growth. That said, there were times when the boys would get into it, and I would reprimand Max. (The whole, *What are you doing to your brother?* Routine.) When, really, Max was trying to help, but Gus would take offense. Max would later come to me and say, "Dad, can we talk? *This* (fill in the blank) is what I was trying to do. I was trying to help him." These kinds of open discussions lead to learning opportunities and learning opportunities lead to growth. Both neurotypical and ASD siblings should have an open environment to discuss their feelings and frustrations. Creating an environment for your children to thrive is key.

In our household, the same rules that applied to Gus applied to Max. We never delineated a punishment that was harsher to one more than the other. But, I think it is safe to say that Max pushed us further over the edge than Gus! Gus, by nature, is a rule follower. Max has always been a rambunctious force of nature and had little issue questioning authority to see just how far he could take a situation. (A born rebel!) Our boys are different from one another, but we love and appreciate their differences. Parenting is never easy, and it gets a bit more difficult with a special needs child. But with patience, teamwork, and a whole lot of focused love, it can be accomplished with success.

I believe that neurotypical siblings learn valuable lessons from their neurodiverse siblings—such as empathy and understanding. Having a sibling with ASD enhances their protective traits as well. When Gus graduated from West Allegheny High School, friends and family were asked to write a letter to the seniors. When every graduate walked off stage, they were handed an envelope with countless letters of love. In Gus's case, all the letters were beautiful, but who wrote the best one? His brother, Mad Max. Max came downstairs, slapped his letter down in front of me, and said, "I am done." It probably took him all of 20 minutes to write his. When he did it so quickly, my first thought was, *Oh, boy. Let me see what he put* ... To my surprise, Max's letter blew away everyone else's:

Gus, I am extremely proud of you. I know you have always wanted to become an architect, and now it's all coming full circle. You clearly have what it takes to become one of the best to ever do it. I will definitely miss you, beyond words. The constant support and advice you've given me has not been taken for granted, even though it may seem like it. I couldn't name one person that has ever disliked you ever. There's a reason for that. I have one of thing to say, one thing that even helps me get through life. Always be yourself. Don't change who you are, I don't care what happens. You are unlike anybody I've ever met, just continue to be yourself.

— Your #1 friend, Max.

It was short but touching. My jock turned into a mix of Oprah Winfrey and Socrates. Michelle and I wept while reading it. (I still get choked up thinking about it.) Max's letter gives me the perfect segue to my next point—appreciate your child.

Autism gave Gus a superpower. As Max alluded to in his letter, Gus looks for the inherent good in people. He is incapable of saying something bad about anyone. Gus radiates positivity and perkiness, which is why I refer to him as my "happy hippie."

People naturally gravitate toward positive people, and both Max's and Gus's friends recognize that quality as one that makes Gus beautifully unique. Max's comments really reflect how Michelle and I always tried to help Gus become the best person he could be. We were never out to change who Gus is at his core. As for Max, he is an exceptional athlete and a powerful young man. He is your proverbial *gym rat* who understands he has to leverage his strength to maximize his performance on the football field. I believe his true strength has been derived from interactions and lessons learned from his brother. Max is a competitor on the field, but a young man who is both protective and empathetic off the field. Football has taught him a number of lessons about discipline, teamwork, responsibility, resilience, and leadership, but Gus has taught him how to be a better human being.

Michelle and I are lucky, having two boys fairly close in age who enjoyed spending a lot of time together. My wife, my parents, or I would take the boys to parks to play on the swings, take them by creek beds to throw rocks (a preferred activity), or watch them ride their scooters or big wheels for hours. The boys spent quality time together, and neither ever felt ignored. Having them together and participating in the same activities fostered a strong bond between them. In fact, Max played a huge role in *overseeing* Gus.

When Max was in middle school, he wanted me to put a basketball hoop in the front yard. Little did I know the impact it would have. All those neighborhood kids from the King Kong swing set days started gravitating back to the house. They would play basketball every single day, to the point they start calling themselves the PBL (Psaros Basketball League).

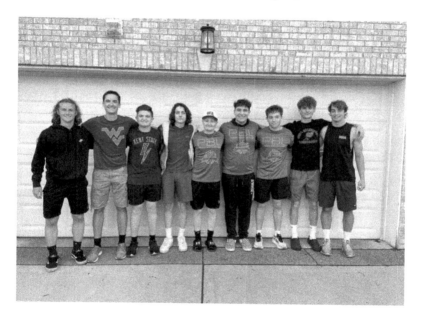

The Psaros Basketball League

The PBL brought together a truly special bunch of young men. All of them are like sons to me. They would show up at our place, blast some rap music, and get down to some hardcore hoopin'. Sure, Gus was a bit hesitant about playing at first. But that didn't matter one bit. The crew welcomed him with open arms. During games, Gus was courtside chatting it up, cheering the guys on, catching up on all the school gossip. Every so often, they'd convince him to get in on the action. This squad was an awesome mix of jocks, band and chorus standouts, and student leaders. Gus needed a village, and you'd be hard pressed to find a better one. He felt comfortable, accepted, and most importantly ... appreciated. Once Max's friends joined the PBL, we would sometimes have upward of 20 to 25 rambunctious young men coming and going from our place. Can you imagine our pizza bill? Eight members of the PBL grew up and graduated high school together. We had a giant photo of them displayed at Gus's high school graduation party held at the Pittsburgh Botanic Garden. Amongst his group of friends, one stands out due to a special connection with Gus: Jakub Stang.

When Gus was in preschool, around the time of his diagnosis, he struggled to socialize with children his own age. However, Michelle noticed a little boy who Gus seemed to gravitate toward. Jakub, known by his Polish nickname, Kuba, was one of four children adopted from Poland. He was, or should I say *is*, a handsome towhead, who, at that time, knew little English.

Picture this: You have a little boy struggling to socialize and gets diagnosed on the spectrum. Then you have another little boy who is trying to learn the English language and assimilate to a completely new life ... and then the two meet. It was like hitting the lottery. Social functioning impairment is a central feature of ASD. Children struggle with eye contact and communication deficits. They get engrossed in their own activities and struggle to understand emotions, so making friends can be quite difficult.

It was a big step for my son to find a friend, and I was moved by it. I will never forget the first time I met Gus's new friend, Jakub. I was walking toward our neighbor's house with Gus on Halloween night when I heard this little voice exclaim, "Gus!" They were instantly two peas in a pod. Seeing my son bond with this adorable little boy was incredible. Until that time, Gus had not truly bonded with any of his peers. In fact, we never saw Gus fully engaged with any of them. With Jakub, Gus was elated to see him, and they immediately had a miraculous bond. It felt like a pair of old souls who knew each other in another life. The dynamic duo ran house to house together, gathering candy, and comparing their loot. It is a moment I will never forget. It was also the first time I was able to meet Jakub's parents, Chris and Dawn—an extraordinary couple that has become a second set of parents to Gus. Jakub's siblings, Oskar, Victoria, and Patryk have been an extension of the family as well. They treat Gus like a sibling.

From that first time I met Jakub, even until now, they've been inseparable. Shortly after they made their connection, Jakob's family moved into our neighborhood, and he has been highly instrumental in Gus's development—he was Gus's gateway into social groups, fashion, and studying sessions ... you name it. I would encourage you to find that one special friend for your child. That one special connection can lead to many more. Friends like Jakub are therapy. Your child is interacting, and the brain is learning from those interactions. If you can find a good friend for your kid, someone who will stand by his or her side, then you are doing OK.

Autism, by default, makes social interactions difficult, so having someone like Jakub to interact with was critical. Because of him, Gus learned to hold a conversation better, read non-verbal cues, including body language and facial expressions, and even maintain eye contact—which was uncomfortable for him at the time. Jakub Stang (the celebrity known as Kuba) proved to us that our son could form meaningful bonds with someone. He quickly became Gus's best friend. It pleases Michelle and me to no end that they remain just as close to this day. Kuba will forever be our third son.

As a parent of an autistic child, helping them make friends can feel daunting, but it is so important for their development. Autistic children often have trouble connecting socially, so we must guide them. It breaks my heart to know that a lot of autistic children celebrate birthdays by themselves or only with family members. With patience and compassion, we can expand their world. When we started PALS, one of the fathers told us how his child had never had a birthday party because he did not have friends. After being a part of the organization, that father told me how he and his wife were able to have three or four kids over and have a meaningful birthday. This is why I strongly suggest parents look into local organizations and centers that feature activities for children on the spectrum. It is not just a great way for parents to develop their village, and meet those other battle-tested parents, but it allows their children to start forming meaningful bonds. When we first founded North Fayette PALS, I mentioned how we were able to meet several incredible families going through the exact same situation. It was not just the parents who were able to find their village, but our children formed bonds from all the structured activities. If one of the children stimmed or had a brief melt down, there was no reason to be embarrassed. All the parents understood it is simply part of ASD.

When it comes to scheduling play dates with other children, whether neurotypical or on the spectrum, observe how your child interacts. (If you schedule a play date with a neurotypical child, start slow.) Before the actual play date, spend some time role playing conversations and teaching your child social cues. If your child is a bit defensive during these discussions, remind them that you are their greatest fan and only there to help. Ideally, your child will be able to develop bonds during play dates, and you can use these play dates as built-in therapy.

Another option is to enroll your child in classes or groups focused on their interests to meet like-minded peers. All interaction is good interaction. (Think of it as "some is better than none.") It is important to celebrate each and every social victory.

If you observe your son or daughter fully engaged with a peer or double the length of a conversation with a friend, show pride and excitement. Guess what? Your child is officially 2% better! The friendship journey may have twists and turns, but you can nurture growth every step of the way. With your support, your child's light will shine through.

I have seen many parents apprehensive about having their child on play dates, taking them to social gatherings, or letting them interact with other children. They keep their child at home, and the child becomes exceptionally isolated. Your child will never get 2% better if they are sitting at home on an electronic device or staring out the window. Friends and siblings matter—they are critical to improving social skills.

Chapter 8: Resilience, Positivity, and Mental Toughness for Parents of Children with Special Needs

"Whoever is happy will make others happy too."[49]

– Anne Frank

Resilience is "an ability to recover from or adjust easily to misfortune or change."[50]

That is the Webster's Dictionary definition, and it's great because it clearly defines what every parent should have for this journey. However, if you are a parent of a child on the spectrum, particularly a father, what you need goes beyond the typical definition of "resilience." There is a particular word that comes to mind. One that is a brilliant representation of what I am talking about.

The Greeks have a word that they own: *philotimo*. It is the most powerful Greek word, and it has no proper definition. *Philotimo* to a Greek is essentially a way of life. Many refer to it as "The Greek Secret." The word comes from the Greek root words "*filos*," which means "friend," and "*timi*," which means "honor." Because there is

---

49 Laura Tscherry, "Anne Frank: 10 beautiful quotes from The Diary of a Young Girl," The Guardian, https://www.theguardian.com/childrens-books-site/2015/jan/27/the-greatest-anne-frank-quotes-ever.
50 Resilience Definition & Meaning. Merriam-Webster. https://www.merriam-webster.com/dictionary/resilience

no true definition, the best way to describe *philotimo* is to think of it in terms of doing good for the sake of doing good. It does not matter how big or small, but it is knowing that an act of kindness has a ripple effect in the universe—you ask nothing in return.

Philotimo encompasses "pride in self, pride in family, pride in community and always doing the right thing."[51] I am hoping this book is a true act of *Philotimo* and is a beacon of light for all fathers with a child on the spectrum.

The Finnish also have a word that they claim as their own; one that is also considered untranslatable. That word is sisu. Sisu is a special strength and persistent resolve to overcome when faced with adversity. It is tenacity of purpose, bravery, grit, and resilience. I think of defining resilience in the terms of the word *sisu*, especially if you have a neurodiverse child, because what you have goes beyond Webster's dictionary definition. It is an undying resilience and refusal to give up fueled by a burning desire to see your child grow and thrive. *Sisu*, to me, is "resilience" on steroids, and I think that is the mentality you need to have as a parent.

It is understanding that you could be at the top of the mountain one day and low in the valley the next. But no matter where you find yourself at the end of the day, you must keep your eye on the prize, fighting for and helping your child.

As explained on the *This is Finland* website, "Etymologically, 'sisu' comes from a Finnish root word that implies 'inner' or

---

[51]Philotimo: A Greek Word Without Meaning but Very Meaningful. (n.d.). Psychology Today. https://www.psychologytoday.com/us/blog/let-their-words-do-the-talking/201508/philotimo-greek-word-without-meaning-very-meaningful

'inside.' For this is one reason it is sometimes translated as 'guts' or 'inner strength'." [52] *Sisu* is not about momentary courage, it is about the ability to sustain that courage. When God hands you a child on the spectrum, I believe He knows He is handing the child to a parent with *sisu* burning in his or her soul. Your job to assist and improve your child is there for life. It is not temporary. The quality of *sisu* I appreciate the most is that people with *sisu* learn from failures and move on. Michelle and I were relentless in our pursuit to assist Gus, and we sustained many failures. Stopping, in frustration, and opting to stagnate was never an option. Parents with children on the spectrum need to learn from a failure, mark it in the "things that did not work" column, and move on.

In previous chapters, we talked about having sight and vision. *Sisu* relates to having vision because you are continually picturing your child at their best. It is embodying unrelenting grit, regardless of what is going on around you. Parents of children on the spectrum need to be beyond resilient. Put it this way, if you were a boxer in the midst of a fight, you would have to keep your guard up. What would happen if you were getting pummeled and dropped your hands? You would get knocked out. You cannot stop in the middle of a fight. You cannot let your guard down—you always have to press forward. I am using one of my favorite motivational speakers and former Green Beret, David Goggins, again to highlight the importance of mindset. Goggins had a horrific childhood and in his book, *Never Finished*, he discusses resilience and bouncing back from his hellish upbringing. The following is an excerpt:

> I adopted a new mindset. I needed to become someone who refused to give in, who simply finds a way no matter what. I needed to become bulletproof, a living example of resilience.

---

[52] Peter Marten. (2018, March 8). The sisu within you: The Finnish key to life, love and success. ThisisFINLAND. https://finland.fi/arts-culture/sisu-within-finnish-key-life-love-success/

Think of a packet of seeds scattered in a garden. Some seeds get more sunlight, more water, and are planted in nourishing topsoil, and because they are put in the right place at the right time, they can rise from seed to seedling to a thriving tree. Seeds planted in too much shade or that don't get enough water may never become anything at all unless someone transplants them—saves them—before it's too late.

Then there are those seedlings that look for the light on their own. They creep from the shade into the sunshine without being transplanted. They find it without anyone digging them up and placing them in the light. They find strength where there is none.

That is resilience.[53]

This excerpt made me think of the resilience required to raise a child on the spectrum. I resonate with Goggins's *no bullshit, no excuses* approach to life. (We live in a society where too many people make too many excuses.) He lives the axiom comfort prevents progression and talks a great deal about the dangers of getting too comfortable. Pause and think about that for a moment. "Comfort prevents progression." If you try one modality, and it fails, what do you do? If your first instinct is to throw your hands up and say, *We're done!* then you have reached comfort mode.

Let's say your child is struggling socially, and group activities are still too overstimulating. Instead of trying out different modalities for interaction with peers to develop their social skills, you may decide to keep your child in the safe harbor of your home.

---

[53] David Goggins, *Never Finished: Unshackle Your Mind and Win the War Within*, (Lioncrest Publishing), 2022, page 32.

Rather than trying something new, or different, to motivate your child to get out and to interact with friends, you opt for the risk-free option. Comfort can actually be detrimental to your child's growth.

While you may think you are helping, I have seen children who essentially become prisoners and almost completely reliant on their parents because the parents have stopped searching for improvement. Your level of resilience needs to be an almost maniacal pursuit of excellence for your child. Can it be disheartening when you come up against a wall? Absolutely, but that is where your inner fighter mentality needs to override discouragement.

I hope you will make the two new words I taught you— *philotimo* and *sisu*—part of your journey. Both are remarkably powerful, and I encourage you to apply both to your daily life. The ultimate act of *philotimo* for me is giving back to the autism community. I strongly encourage you to get involved, share your knowledge, and most importantly, help others. Some choose to do little in life, while others believe in making an impact. Be the beacon of light that shines through darkness. To quote Jackie Robinson, "A life is not important except in the impact it has on other lives."[54] *Sisu* is within every parent with a child or children on the spectrum. Tap into this special power. Use it to make your children the best that they can be. God chose you for a reason. Never take that for granted. He saw your *inner sisu*. Use your superpower to help your child grow.

Right around when Gus was diagnosed, Michelle and I had to deal with a lot of snake-oil salesmen. We would get our hopes up

---

[54] Jackie Robinson, Goodreads, https://www.goodreads.com/quotes/38636-a-life-is-not-important-except-in-the-impact-it.

and try a supplement, only to find out that it did not work. But we did not let that deter us—we never stopped looking for modalities that would help our son. The most difficult scenario, for me, was an experience we had with a physician who wrote an utterly fascinating book. It was a paradigm shift of thinking. Even the physician's title of the book was controversial, but he framed autism in a new light. He introduced me to the NeuroSPECT scan. According to Mayo Clinic, a NeuroSPECT is a test that creates a detailed, 3D map of the blood flow activity in your brain, which can be helpful in determining which parts of the brain need enhanced.[55]

The pandemic in 2020 freed up a lot of my time, and I was able to read the book for a second time. I spoke with Michelle, and we agreed to reach out to the physician's office. (Michelle was a saint. She had to fill out an inordinate amount of paperwork to get established with his practice!) This doctor was on the west coast, and we would have to complete all our visits virtually. We were filled with hope that this physician and his new approach would be life-altering for Gus. Things did *not* go as planned.

From the very first exorbitantly expensive virtual call, we started to question if we made the right move. This physician came across as eccentric, possibly a quack. He decided that half of the call would be a bizarre political commercial while the other half would be about Gus's situation. After our first virtual visit, he immediately prescribed Gus a selective serotonin reuptake inhibitor (SSRI) that caused him to gain weight (between 15 to 20 pounds). Each appointment seemed to be a greater waste of time. The physician would spend more time ranting about the recent presidential election and less time on my son.

---

[55] Mayo Clinic Staff, Mayo Clinic, https://www.mayoclinic.org/tests-procedures/spect-scan/about/pac-20384925.

Michelle and I desperately wanted a NeuroSPECT scan of our son's brain, but we had to comply with the physician's leisurely process. On the fourth call with the physician, once again, he started by ranting about politics. Michelle jumped up from the call and simply walked away. She, like me, had simply had enough.

I stopped the physician and bluntly stated, "Doctor, I do not care if your candidate lost the presidential election. I am tired of listening to rants about recounts—I want to hear about my son." The call proceeded, but I could tell he was not pleased with my comment. That was the final call we ever made to the physician.

Michelle and I had wasted time, spent an exorbitant amount of money, and added weight to Gus's midsection. Nothing positive or productive came from the experience. Although we felt swindled, we never looked at each other and stated, *That is it!* We are done. While we might have been done with that particular physician, we never gave up on seeking new modalities. We experienced a sizeable failure, but our *sisu* level of determination kept us pursuing improvement. I still have the NeuroSPECT scan in the back of my pocket and plan on finding a physician and medical facility that will work with us. Giving up on the process would essentially be giving up on our son ... and that wasn't an option.

Raising a child on the spectrum can be difficult, but remember, God chose you for this monumental, yet beautiful task. Parents can face many hardships, especially in their relationships. (Remember the scenario of rowing the boat? If you are both rowing in the same direction, the boat takes off.) The stress and overwhelm that comes with this blessed assignment can be detrimental to your health and well-being if you do not get it under control. This is why there is one other factor that I want to touch on before I end this chapter because I think it is vitally important: positivity.

Resilience and positivity go hand in hand. If you ask my wife what my favorite song is, she'll tell you it is Monty Python's, "Always Look on The Bright Side of Life." (Well, that, followed by 20 heavy metal songs.) Not only was Monty Python the greatest comedy troop of all time, but they were also brilliant at analyzing life's journey. In their song, the lyrics state:

Some things in life are bad
They can really make you mad
Other things just make you swear and curse
When you're chewing on life's gristle
Don't grumble, give a whistle
And this'll help things turn out for the best
And ... Always look on the bright side of life[56]

I do not do negative. I am just not wired for it. I have covered University of Pittsburgh sports now for over 25 years, and I am known as the amplifier—Mr. Positivity. I know what you are thinking, *OK, Mr. Happy. You do not have a bad day?*

Of course, I do. My wife and I experienced exceptionally difficult times. We have been knocked down time and time again. The key to not letting it keep you down is to redirect your mindset. I always found time for self-care. I went for a quick run, read a chapter in a book, hit the heavy bag or the gym, or smiled and refocused.

For my wife, she squeezed in a workout, did yoga, or hung out at a bookstore (her favorite). Without self-care and positivity, you are sunk. A positivity mindset is your biggest superpower—it needs to be your steady state. When you are around someone who is

---

[56] Eric Idle, vocalist, "Always Look on The Brightside of Life," Andre Jacquemin and Dave Howman (producers), 1979.

positive, there is energy in the room. It is tangible. I believe that it is infectious.

When someone radiates positivity, it rubs off on you. You feel your spirits lift simply by being around a positive person, and it's like you are literally being recharged.

Unfortunately, the brain has a built-in negative bias. That means your brain will naturally focus on negativity and bad things. However, I believe in the concept of neuroplasticity; the brain *can* synaptically change. I have seen it firsthand in my son through the Brain Balance concept, rewiring the brain.

If you are the parent of a child with ASD, in particular, a father, you need to do a gut check and reframe your mindset. (Dads, you are the leader of your village—there is zero wiggle room for negativity!) If you feel that you tend to dwell on the negative, or maybe have not been a resilient parent, you can change. It all starts with focusing on the day-to-day. I want you to think about all that you are asking of your child—you are asking him or her to change. Let me ask you, *What do they see when they look at you?*

Your 2% improvement is no different. Set the example. You can work toward building positivity and resilience. Consistent negativity does *nothing* for you, your marriage, or—most importantly—the development of your child. Complaints, arguments, and yelling are all toxins that poison a household. (If negativity has a stronghold on you, and you are really struggling, please see my contact information at the end of the book. I believe that you, too, can change!) Maintaining a positive mindset is healthier for everyone.

Do not get me wrong, positive people do have negative moments, but the difference is how they respond. Resilience allows them to reframe their mindset and think, *You know what? I am going to stop right here. This sucks right now, but tomorrow is going to be better.* They are painting that mental picture, which can be a motivational pause. When you are positive, you are setting the standard, which spreads to other family members.

I believe positive people bring unique perspectives to problems. They hold on to the belief that there is a solution to every problem— even if the problem is remarkably difficult. This mindset allows them to look at long-term outcomes and envision the best-case scenario. This is where the vision piece we previously talked about comes into play.

Not every day is going to be perfect, far from it. Children on the spectrum and their family members are by default going to struggle. However, the struggle will eventually lead to somewhere better, regardless of where your child is on the spectrum.

If you are having an exceptionally shitty day, think about where you are going. If your child hits a roadblock, focus on your vision because that will reframe the image. (Remember the smile rule? Think to yourself, *This too shall pass. I am ready for tomorrow.*)

If you are a father, you are also a teacher, and you are there to leave a legacy. I would encourage you to create a healthy, positive environment in your household and never lose hope for your child because they are depending on you. I often think about what my boys will think of me. If they look back and say, *Dad was really a negative guy*, I've done something wrong. One of the biggest factors in why I do not do negative is a testament to my parents, Mary Ann and George.

Everybody has ups and downs, but my brother, Mike, and I are wired for hope and positivity. All that goes back to parenting. Again, if you are the father and are leading the pack, negativity and toxicity set the worst examples. What does toxicity look like? There are different facets to this. If one spouse is constantly complaining, denying the diagnosis, or throwing out comments that this is *someone's fault*, the child's progress will be stunted. I have seen this firsthand time and time again.

The parent who is the denier is like an anchor thrown overboard from a ship. Once the anchor locks into the ocean floor, that ship cannot progress. What happens to the parent who is on board? The one trying to be positive and help? They get burnt out really quickly. Even if both parents are on board, the complaints, arguments, and yelling make the environment toxic. In a household, you need the collective energy to be positive and to tackle each day. Yes, you will run into problems, and that can be frustrating, but you all need to be unified in purpose. And if you go into any situation with a positive, constructive mindset, life is a hell of a lot better and a hell of a lot easier.

If you start to bicker and argue or are thinking your child is going to improve overnight, then it becomes a long slog. If you start yelling at your child, you will significantly hinder your child's progress and disrupt your entire family. You need patience ... and patience is a big word!

Again, the life of a parent with one or more children with ASD is not all sunshine and roses; the angels are not singing over you every day. Arguments happen, especially if both parents are exhausted— we are all just human at the end of the day. But if you both, as parents, constantly chide each other or complain, especially about the time and effort needed for your child's improvement, it will stress out your child. If you are complaining about sitting in traffic for an hour to *drive to damn therapy again* after working a full day, that weighs on a child, especially if the child is mild. They have an awareness, and they could start to believe that they are causing all the problems. If Michelle's perspective of therapy was, *That is it! My day is done. I can't get to yoga because I have to go to therapy, and we will not get back until 10 at night!* we would have hit a brick wall.

Nonstop complaining does nothing but emit negativity and toxicity into a house. Insinuating that autism is bad by blaming every problem on it, punishing your child for stimming or melting down, or trying to *cure* your child (Remember, the goal is to improve, not cure!) is especially harmful to children with autism because they have sensory issues. So, when someone yells, the amplified voice triggers their fight or flight mechanism, and these children stop listening. Parents who yell the most are heard the least. Avoid all these negative behaviors. Be a beacon of light instead.

I know what some of you may be thinking as you read this: *Enough with the psychobabble already! There is zero evidence that starting each day with a sunny disposition will actually improve my difficult situation.* I understand your skepticism. When life feels overwhelmingly difficult, suggestions to *look on the bright side* can ring hollow, but hear me out. Before you completely write me off, consider the cultural force of the television show, *Ted Lasso.*[57] In 2020, the show became a true phenomenon.

The brilliant Jason Sudeikis plays the title character, Ted Lasso. Ted is a college football coach who is hired to coach the ragtag English Premier League soccer team, AFC Richmond essentially because the owner wants the ultimate revenge on her ex-husband: to run the team he used to own into the ground. The whole premise of the show is that they hire Ted Lasso as the coach because they think he is an incompetent rube from the States. However, through

---

[57] Hunt, B., Kelly, J., Lawrence, B., Sudeikis, J., Waddingham, H., & Swift, J. (2020, August 14). Ted Lasso. IMDb. https://www.imdb.com/title/tt10986410/?ref_=fn_al_tt_1

his optimism, positivity, and ability to lift others' spirits, he elevates the entire franchise.

Ted Lasso is more than just a feel-good show. It is a masterclass in leadership and human connection. With his unwavering optimism and compassion, the mustachioed coach breathes new life into a struggling football club. He does not berate or bully his team—Ted chooses empathy over ego, and his players respond. They rally around this man who believes in them when they do not believe in themselves. Ted reminds us that being kind and lifting others up is a leader's greatest strength. His infectious positivity transforms not just a team, but an entire community.

The show illuminates how powerful it is to lead with love and how nurturing the human spirit bears more fruit than crushing it. Ted calls us to choose gentleness over harshness and to see the humanity in each other. The revolution he sparked is one we desperately need.

Ted Lasso does not just charm viewers with its heartwarming story—it changes the game for leadership, coaching, and most importantly, parenting. Experts have dubbed it the "Ted Lasso effect."[58] The show imparts timeless wisdom that can enrich our lives, like believing in yourself even when no one else does; having the courage to try, fail, and try again; seeing the good in others; and meeting them where they are. Also, vulnerability does not make you weak; it makes you human. Tell the truth but lead with compassion. Winning is a mindset, not an outcome. Stay curious and grow every

---

[58] Anthony Martin, "The Ted Lasso Effect: Cultural Collisions, Sport, and the Rise of the Human Story," Greenbook, July 6, 2023,

https://www.greenbook.org/insights/research-methodologies/the-ted-lasso-effect-cultural-collisions-sport-and-the-rise-of-the-human-story#.

day. If you make a mistake, forgive yourself quickly (like a goldfish), then keep swimming.

Ted reminds us that happiness is a choice. His infectious optimism lifts up every person he meets. With open arms, he embraces the unique gifts in each of his players. He knows that when you do the right thing, it's never wrong. In a cynical world, Ted is a ray of hope. His wisdom can make us all a little better if we dare to lead with heart. Though life brings sorrow, there is still profound joy to be found. The lasting impact of this show proves it.

So, what does this have to do with autism? The show captures hearts for its simple yet profound wisdom. As a parent of a child on the autism spectrum, I have found the show's lessons to be deeply resonant. I know firsthand how challenging, yet rewarding this journey can be. But in times of doubt and frustration, a show like *Ted Lasso* teaches us to lead with kindness. Though the days are long, and progress can feel slow, Ted teaches us that positivity is contagious. With empathy and understanding, we, as parents, allow our children to truly see themselves through our eyes. We become their mirror.

Creating a culture of happiness at home nurtures growth for your child on the spectrum. Your child's daily progress depends on the environment you cultivate. Like seeds in fertile soil, children blossom when given warmth, patience, and encouragement. But stress, conflict, and anger stunt their development. By fostering joy and compassion within your family, you help your child reach their full potential. With mindfulness and unity, your home can be a greenhouse where your child flourishes.

This reflection goes both ways. Our children have so much to show us if we take the time to listen and learn how to have patience, acceptance, and live in the present. Our children illuminate the path. Together, we can create a nurturing environment where our children are free to grow into their fullest selves. Where patience and compassion bloom. Where differences are celebrated. Where love and light shine brighter than any challenge that threatens to dim our spirit along the way.

Gus embodies many of the same values, day after day. These lessons have permeated my very DNA, as Ted might say. Gus teaches me to be truer to myself and find joy in each moment. For that, I'm forever grateful.

Let me expound on four *Ted Lasso* lessons that Gus exemplifies daily:

1. **See the good in others.** Gus possesses a remarkable gift that we could all learn from. His autism allows him to see only the good in people, making it impossible for him to speak ill of anyone. What an incredible superpower! Whenever I am with Gus, I am reminded of humanity's boundless potential for kindness. His gentle spirit and unwavering optimism humble me. He looks past flaws and finds the light in everyone, even when they cannot see it themselves. The world would certainly be a warmer, more loving place if we all shared Gus's special talent. He inspires me to search for the good in people and focus less on judgment. We have much to learn from such a pure heart.

2. **Courage is about being willing to try.** Gus understands what true courage is. It is not about being fearless, but being willing to try even when you are afraid. He has faced so many challenges that pushed him outside his comfort zone, experiences that did not come naturally to someone on the autism spectrum. Public speaking that made his heart race. Social interactions that felt utterly foreign. Advocating for himself at school despite the anxiety. Attempting sports while dealing with overwhelming sensory issues. None of it was easy,

yet Gus always kept an open mind, and he never stopped trying. He learned and grew from each experience, no matter how uncomfortable it was.

Gus knows that is where real courage lies—in facing the fear. His perseverance in the face of such difficulties is inspiring. It shows the depths of his inner strength and heart.

3. **Optimists do more.** (My favorite) Let me repeat, optimists do more. If there is one iconic image and saying from *Ted Lasso* that will resonate in perpetuity, it will be the simple yet powerful one-word mantra, "Believe." Even if you have never seen the show, you've undoubtedly seen the image: bright yellow rectangular background with a simplistic blue "Believe" written on top. Gus is the embodiment of optimism—a shining light that radiates belief. His path has been far from easy; nothing has fallen perfectly into place. Yet he persists, propelled by a boundless optimism deep in his soul. While the world sees obstacles, Gus sees opportunity. Autism has not defined his limits, only his possibilities. He blazes forward with quiet confidence, never complaining or choosing negativity. He simply believes: in himself, in his gifts, in the plan God has written for him. Belief is Gus's superpower. With it, he can accomplish anything. Just like Ted Lasso might say, *optimism begets action.* When we believe, we do more. Gus lives this truth every day. His light reminds us to have faith in ourselves, in each other, and in life. Anything is possible when we believe.

4. **Happiness is a choice.** To quote the Joker in the movie *The Dark Knight*, "Why so serious?"[59] Happiness awaits those who seek it. Why walk around with a frown when you can greet

---

[59] The Dark Knight (2008) - IMDb. (n.d.). Www.imdb.com. https://www.imdb.com/title/tt0468569/characters/nm0005132

each day with a smile? Take it from Gus, who wakes up each morning bursting with joy. His cheerful, "Hi Dad!" lifts my spirits, proving that an upbeat attitude is contagious. Yes, life has its challenges; even the happiest people in life have bad days. But staying positive helps you weather the storms. Anger and bitterness will only drag you down. If you are consistently angry, complaining, and argumentative, do not blame others or your situation, blame yourself. The person in the mirror has a daily choice—choose to be a ray of light for those around you. The power lies within! You can turn your outlook around in an instant. Will you wallow in gloom or radiate light? Heed the wisdom of Emerson, "For every minute you are angry you lose sixty seconds of happiness."[60] Seize the day! Spread sunshine! *Why so serious, my friends?* Happiness awaits!

Gus personifies these four lessons; however, I think if *anyone* embodied these four principles, they would live a better life. Negativity spreads quickly throughout a household. It is the path of least resistance, and, unfortunately, humans often default to this state. Do you really want your child to replicate your negativity? How will that help his or her progress? I strongly suggest you set them up for positivity instead. Your children learn from you. Children on the spectrum are often asked to deliver 100% effort (maybe more) to improve 2% each day.

When parents join forces with their child's support team, it can truly make a difference. I define your child's support team as anyone in a position to assist your child, such as speech-language pathologists, occupational therapists, teachers, physical therapists, audiologists, paraprofessionals, neurologists, and developmental

---

[60] A quote by Ralph Waldo Emerson. (n.d.). Www.goodreads.com. https://www.goodreads.com/quotes/353-for-every-minute-you-are-angry-you-lose-sixty-seconds

and behavioral pediatricians. By collaborating with these professionals, families help create a unified front that allows their child to thrive. Regular, positive communication ensures everyone is on the same page regarding goals, strategies, and progress. With teamwork and understanding, they pave the path for growth and success.

I once spoke with a mother who had a son on the spectrum. He was attending a local high school, and the mother started our conversation with a prolonged series of complaints. Her negative energy was palpable. She then told me about how she interacted with her son's therapists, teachers, and paraprofessionals.

The mother wagged her finger in my face, then emphatically stated, "I believe the squeaky wheel is heard the most. I have little issue demanding what I want for my son. I don't let up." Ten minutes into her diatribe, I interrupted and asked, "So, how is this approach working?"

She indicated that she felt resistance from all of them, some were slow to respond to her requests (demands), and her frustrations were growing exponentially. I did not want to overstep, but I reminded her that she was taking a confrontational and negative tone with people in place to assist her son. Perhaps stepping back, recognizing that they are working together as a team and re-focusing everyone's attention on her son's goals would be the best approach. Nobody wants to work with someone who is caustic and hostile. Remember what I said about our default state, *Negativity is the path of least resistance.* Resist it!

I understand that, in some cases, you may have issues with school districts and outside professionals, and you have to be a bit more forceful with them. But in general, a good rule is to remember all these people are trying to help your child. You will achieve optimal outcomes if you work *with* them. Why take on a threatening or negative tone? Being belligerent does not accomplish anything. Effective partnerships between you and your child's support team are essential. As parents, Michelle and I have always aimed to cultivate a collaborative relationship with Gus's care team by expressing gratitude, empathy, and mutual respect. Though challenging at times, focusing on open communication and shared goals allowed us to build trust and work together as allies. Maintaining positive relationships with providers strengthens the care network and improves quality of life for the entire family.

Bottom line: children with ASD and their parents are dealing with a multitude of people in their care journey, and being kind goes a long way.

Will you and your child see all these people at once? No, but you will see many of them on a weekly basis, and if you are treating all these people like garbage, they will not want to see you. You do not want to be that family where the professionals think, *Here we go*, when you book an appointment or walk into the room. When I talk about toxicity, it does not just apply at home. Creating an adversarial environment does not help your child improve. In fact, it creates undo stress and tension.

Your child's support team likely includes even more than the list of professionals I already mentioned. It can also include a behavior specialist, mobile therapist, specialty trained staff support person, various physicians, possibly a physician assistant or nurse practitioner, relationship development intervention (RDI) professional, play therapist (WonderKids fell into this category), cognitive-behavioral therapist, and music therapist. You are dealing with a collective team, and they are all there to help. In the last four to six years, I've seen the degradation of manners in society. Do not be part of that trend.

Being negative and combative inhibits the rapport you need to have with these individuals. You can be a "squeaky wheel," and still be tactful. Work *with* these professionals: listen to them, thank them, and do not forget that you are all a part of your child's team. In the words of Hellen Keller, "Alone we can do so little, together we can do so much."[61]

If you get nothing else from reading this book, I hope you realize the importance of these two words: *positivity* and *resilience*. Make them your mantra. Hell, make them part of your DNA. Remember, positivity is a mindset, and children on the autism spectrum often respond well to positive reinforcement. Praise them for doing well. If they do something wrong, do not snap at them or say things like, *No! You did that wrong.* Instead, consider phrases like, *What if we did it like this instead?* Stay consistent, on a schedule, and as patient as possible. Not every modality, treatment, or approach will work with your child, but instead of complaining and having a meltdown, think of it as one step closer to finding the next modality that works. I could go on forever, but how it goes comes down to mindset.

---

[61] Helen Keller Quotes on Progress | American Foundation for the Blind. https://www.afb.org/about-afb/history/helen-keller/helen-keller-quotes/helen-keller-quotes-progress

Chapter 9: Warrior Parents: Navigating the Battlefield with Unyielding Love

"Let perseverance be your engine and hope your fuel."[62]

– H. Jackson Brown, Jr.

There are moments in life that can catch you by surprise. I entered a rare open weekend that ended up etched in my memory. As Michelle and I tackled the mountain of chores awaiting us, I stumbled upon a Rocky movie marathon playing on TV, and it was just what I needed to power through the cleaning. I watched each film with bated breath as Rocky triumphed over one daunting foe after another—the flashy Apollo Creed, the menacing Clubber Lang, the icy Ivan Drago and his venomous wife, and the arrogant Tommy Gunn. By the sixth installment, *Rocky Balboa*, I was ready to switch it off, exhausted from the day's work. But then came a favorite scene of mine. It shook me to my core and left me transfixed. A simple, yet profound moment that spoke to the heart of Rocky's underdog journey (the one I shared with Gus). I will never forget the surge of inspiration that coursed through me in that instant:

Let me tell you something you already know. The world ain't all sunshine and rainbows. It's a very mean and nasty place and I don't care how tough you are, it will beat you to your knees and

---

[62] H. Jackson Brown, JR. quotes and sayings.
https://www.inspiringquotes.us/author/3878-h-jackson-brown-jr

keep you there permanently if you let it. You, me, or nobody is gonna hit as hard as life. But it ain't about how hard you hit. It's about how hard you can get hit and keep moving forward. How much you can take and keep moving forward. That's how winning is done![63]

That small soliloquy Stallone's character gives his son about grit and life being tough is such a passionate scene. I was intently listening as Stallone was getting choked up delivering this speech, and thought, *Holy hell! This is the whole premise of my book!* What a brilliant quote about resilience and grit—especially coming through someone with a boxing background. The end is a perfect positive message: *That is how winning is done.* It is everything I want a father with a child on the spectrum to walk away with; It's the perfect mindset.

When you receive the news that your child is on the autism spectrum, it feels like the wind has been knocked out of you. The road ahead seems daunting and filled with challenges that you may not feel equipped to handle. But take heart. This child has been gifted to you for a reason. God saw the resilience within you, the tenderness in your soul, and knew you were the perfect parent for this exceptional journey.

There will be hard days ahead. Days where you feel defeated and want to give up, but remember this: *You were chosen.* You have been entrusted with this precious child because you have the spirit to weather the storms. You will find strength you never knew you had. Your capacity to love will deepen in ways you cannot yet imagine.

---

[63] Rocky Balboa (2006) - IMDb. (n.d.).
https://www.imdb.com/title/tt0479143/characters/nm0000230

This is not a curse, but a blessing. Embrace it with arms wide open.

Meet each new obstacle with courage, armed with faith in your abilities. You and your child will climb mountains together. Keep your gaze upward and step forward with hope. This path has twists and turns, but I hope sharing our story will help you will navigate yours with wisdom and grace. Your child is a gift, and so are you.

As we near the end of our journey together, I want to emphasize some of the key lessons we have covered throughout these chapters that can help you thrive as a parent of an autistic child.

Firstly, you need to support your spouse wholeheartedly and make sure you are aligned on the goals and visions for your child's future. Think back to my boat rowing analogy, if you are rowing in different directions, you will never move forward. Both you and your spouse must be passionate about your child's potential and have faith that small, daily improvements can lead to enormous growth over time. This step is essential for your child's betterment. Next, you will need to build a strong village of support around your family—make sure to include and empower siblings and friends to rally around your child and do their own research. Then, make sure to take exquisite care of yourself. You are leading by example so your children will learn self-care. Even though you have a busy schedule, and the days are long, this needs to be a priority. Unless you take care of yourself first, you cannot expect to show up and care for others.

You also must remember that your child with autism needs both sight and vision. Sight is living in the present—supporting your child's daily growth and development. Vision is the big picture—your long-term hopes and dreams for your child. Keeping both in constant focus is key to staying on track. With sight, celebrate each new milestone achieved. With vision, plant seeds today that will blossom into the life you envision for your child. When you balance the now and the someday, you will guide your child on a meaningful journey filled with purpose, growth, and joy.

Lastly, no matter how difficult the path may seem at times, stay relentlessly positive and resilient. You need to model hope and determination in the face of challenges for your child; he or she will need it. If you keep these core principles at the heart of your parenting, you can unlock your child's potential while creating deeper connections and joy within your family. The journey is not easy, but it is so worth it.

Throughout this book I have attempted to share useful information. Let me flip the script with one final request. I implore you to be a force for good. Your voice and passion are needed. We stand at a critical moment in time. With each passing day, more children receive an autism diagnosis; more parents have their lives forever altered by a few words. These families need you—your wisdom, empathy, and tested experience. You have the power to lift them up during their darkest hours. So, I urge you to take these words to heart, feel their weight, and let them move you to action. Lend your light to those traversing this difficult path, so that no one walks alone. Together, we can build a community of care, compassion, and hope. Our hands can steady families when they feel unmoored. Our voices can guide them forward. If we link arms, we can change lives. The time for action is now. The families need you. The children need you. Let me repeat what I consistently tell my sons, "In life, you're either sitting on the bench or you're playing in the game." I implore all of you to be an MVP.
I want to thank you for reading this book. There is an abundance of books on treatments and therapies, and I wanted to avoid writing the latest because every child and every plan is highly individualized. This is a journey of the heart—one we walk together, hand in hand. I do not know how much of this journey resonated with you, but my hope is that you found comfort, wisdom, and

inspiration in these pages. Whether you're just starting your journey with autism or have been on this path for a while, please know that your mindset matters deeply. My hope is that this book ignited a spark of hope, positivity, and resilience within you. Your child is your purpose. Like Benjamin Disraeli said, "Nothing can resist a human will that will stake its very existence on its purpose."[64] You have the power to shape your child's future. So let your will be strong, your purpose be true, and your heart be open. Together, we will elevate autism one beautiful mind at a time.

To all you warrior moms and dads out there, let these words seep into your soul and ignite your inner fire: I see your strength. I see your courage. I see your unbreakable spirit. You walk this path not for yourself, but for your child who depends on you. Though there are days of darkness and frustration, you shine as a beacon of hope. You are a light in the shadows. An anchor in the storm. You are the calm in the midst of chaos. So, lift your head high, press your shoulders back, and pick your chin up. Make your stance wide and sturdy. Plant your feet firmly and stand tall because you are a protector, a nurturer, and guardian of all that is good.

Within you burns a warrior's heart—unyielding, unafraid, unstoppable. This is your time to rise, take up arms, link shields, and unite as one. You, remarkable parent, are stronger than you know. You are greater than any challenge you will face, so believe in yourself. Have faith in your power, go forth boldly, and give 'em hell.

---

[64] Quote by Benjamin Disraeli: "Nothing can resist a human will that will stake..." Goodreads. https://www.goodreads.com/quotes/9995019-nothing-can-resist-a-human-will-that-will-stake-its

About the Author

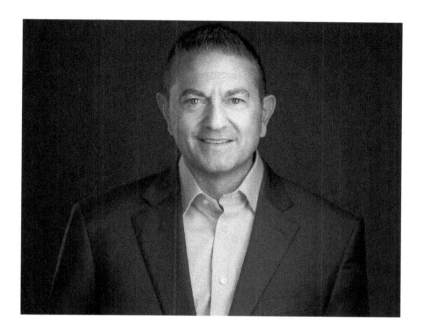

A devoted family man, Harry Psaros has been happily married to his wife Michelle for 24 years and is a proud father of two sons, Costa ("Gus") and Maximos ("Max"). Originally from the steel town of Weirton, W.Va., Psaros has called McDonald, Pa., home for the past two decades.

Professionally, Psaros serves as an executive neuroscience account specialist for AbbVie. He is on the board of directors for the Autism Caring Center, one of the founders of North Fayette P.A.L.S. (an organization for special needs children), president of North Fayette Township's parks and recreation board, and vice president of All Saints Greek Orthodox Church in Weirton, W.Va. Known affectionately by fans as the "Pitt Guru," he is a top social media influencer for University of Pittsburgh athletics and the senior writer for *Pittsburgh Sports Now*.

With a bachelor of science in industrial engineering from the University of Pittsburgh, as well as minors in physics and philosophy, Psaros has a strong educational foundation. Further expanding his expertise, he obtained a certification as a health coach from the Institute of Integrated Nutrition.

Harry is an avid reader, enjoys strength training, running, and martial arts and lives to serve others. He believes that "if you are breathing air, you should be helping others."

Contact Harry

Websites: StruggletoStrength.org

HarryPsaros.com

LinkedIn: Harry Psaros

Email: harrypsaros2828@gmail.com

Facebook: Harry Psaros

X: @PittGuru

TikTok: @harrypsaros

www.ingramcontent.com/pod-product-compliance
Lightning Source LLC
Chambersburg PA
CBHW051919020225
21234CB00003B/11